CHAIR YOGA FOR SENIORS TO LOSE WEIGHT

Unlocking Weight Loss Potential with Gentle 10 Minutes Exercises for Rapid Results and Improved Mobility with 28-Days Challenge.

Daniel S. Leeper

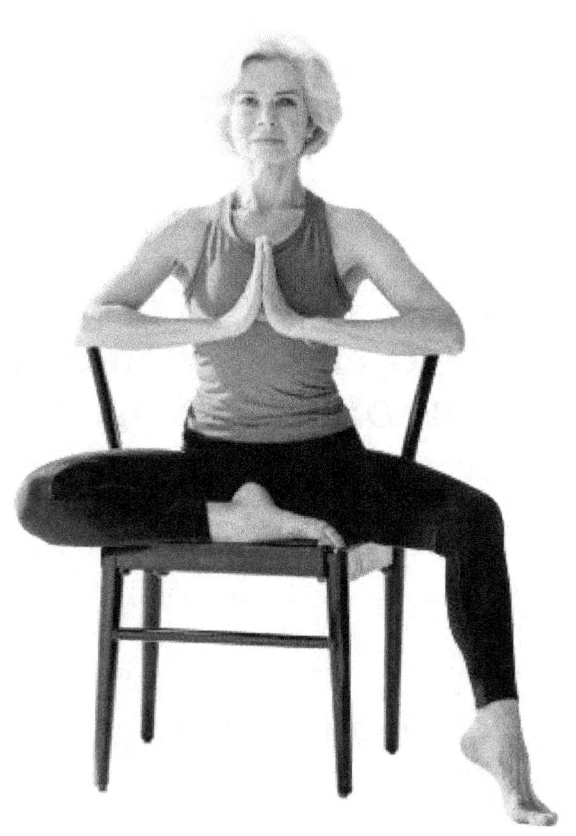

Table of Contents

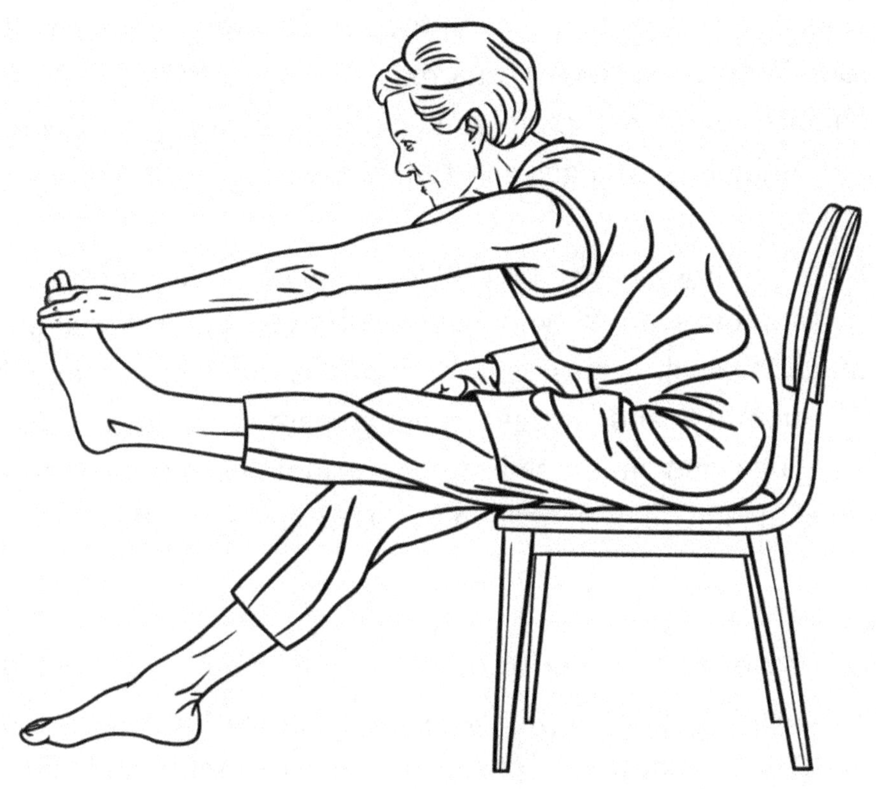

Introduction

In this comprehensive guide, we'll delve into the transformative power of chair yoga for seniors seeking to shed unwanted pounds and reclaim their vitality.

As a professional fitness coach, I've witnessed the remarkable benefits of chair yoga for seniors. While traditional yoga may seem daunting for those with limited mobility or balance concerns, chair yoga offers a gentle yet effective alternative accessible to individuals of all ages and fitness levels.

Throughout my journey as a fitness coach, I've witnessed incredible transformations among seniors who have embraced chair yoga as part of their wellness routine. One such inspiring story involves my dear auntie, who, like many seniors, faced mobility and weight management challenges. By consistently practising chair yoga and implementing the principles outlined in this book, she shed excess weight and experienced newfound strength, flexibility, and overall well-being.

But my auntie's story is just one example among many. I've had the honour of working with numerous older adults who have reaped the rewards of chair yoga, achieving weight loss, improved posture, reduced stress, and enhanced mental clarity. Their success stories testify to the transformative potential of chair yoga for seniors.

Inside this book, you'll discover a wealth of information, including the science behind chair yoga's impact on weight loss, practical tips for getting started, various chair yoga poses tailored specifically for seniors, and strategies for incorporating chair yoga into your daily routine.

Whether you're a seasoned yogi or a complete beginner, "Chair Yoga for Seniors to Lose Weight" is your roadmap to a healthier, more vibrant life. Join me on this journey as we unlock the secret to sustainable weight loss and embrace a lifestyle of health, happiness, and fulfilment.

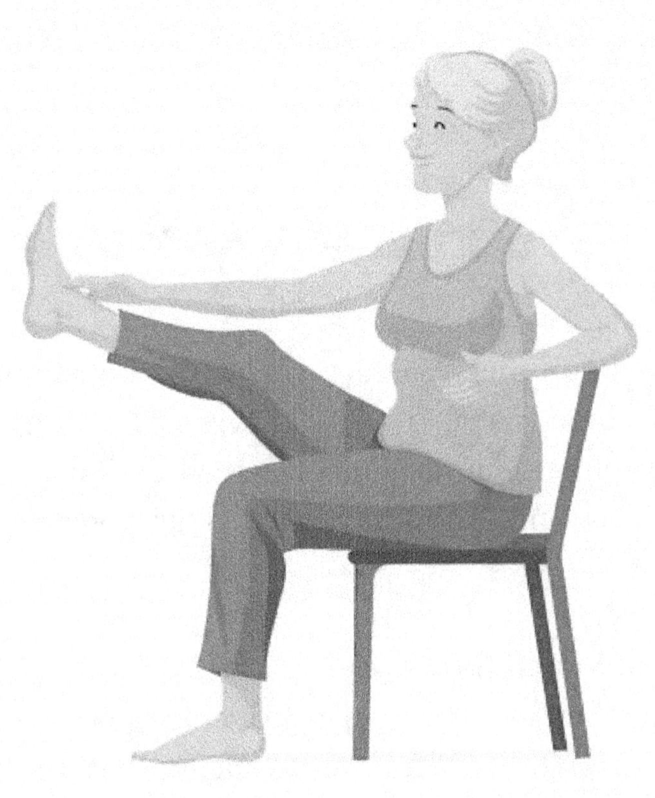

Chapter 1: Benefits of Chair Yoga for Seniors

In this chapter, we'll look at the several benefits that chair yoga provides seniors trying to enhance their health and well-being, specifically emphasizing how it can help with weight loss.

1.1 An Introduction to Chair Yoga for Seniors

Staying active as we age is increasingly vital for maintaining our general health and mobility. On the other hand, traditional types of exercise can be difficult or even impossible for seniors due to variables such as joint discomfort, decreased mobility, or balance concerns. This is where chair yoga excels as a gentle yet effective option.

Improves mobility and flexibility.
One of the key benefits of chair yoga for elders is increased mobility and flexibility. Many chair yoga postures are meant to gently stretch and strengthen muscles, ligaments, and joints, allowing seniors to maintain or enhance their range of motion. This enhanced mobility improves daily functioning while lowering the chance of falls and accidents.

Gentle Stretching to Improve Flexibility
Gentle stretching is an important part of chair yoga since it improves flexibility, promotes joint health, and relieves muscular tension. Unlike more strenuous types of exercise that may damage ageing bodies, chair yoga stretches are deliberate and controlled, providing a safe and effective method of increasing flexibility without generating undue stress or discomfort.

Understanding The Physiology of Stretching

Before diving into specific chair yoga poses, it's useful to understand how stretching works and why it's so important for keeping flexibility, especially as we get older. Whether in chair yoga or other modalities, stretching movements work the muscles, tendons, and connective tissues that surround and support our joints.

As we stretch these tissues, they gradually elongate and become more flexible, allowing for a wider range of motion in the joints. This improved flexibility allows us to move more freely and minimizes the chance of injury by improving joint stability and resiliency. Stretching also increases blood flow to the muscles, supplying essential nutrients and oxygen while eliminating toxins and metabolic waste products.

Key Principles for Gentle Stretching in Chair Yoga

Chair yoga focuses on gentle, controlled motions that gradually coax the body into deeper stretches over time. Seniors are advised to move thoughtfully, focusing on their breath and any feelings during the stretch. Stretching must be approached with patience and compassion, considering the body's limitations and avoiding pain or discomfort.

Various stretching techniques can be used in chair yoga to target certain muscle groups and parts of the body. Some typical ways include static stretching (holding a stretch for an extended time) and dynamic stretching (moving through a range of motion in a controlled manner).

Chair Yoga Poses: Gentle Stretching

Now, let's look at some chair yoga positions meant to encourage gentle stretching and better flexibility in seniors:

1. Seated Forward Fold: Start sitting erect on your chair, feet flat on the floor. Inhale to stretch the spine, then exhale as you bend forward from the hips and reach your hands toward your feet or the floor. Keep your back straight and avoid rounding the spine. Hold a few breaths and feel your hamstrings and lower back stretch.

2. Seated Side Stretch: Sit comfortably in your chair, feet hip-width apart. Inhale to stretch your spine, then exhale while reaching one arm overhead and leaning gently to the other side. Keep both sit bones on the chair to avoid collapsing into the stretch. Hold for a few breaths, and then switch sides.

3. Seated Spinal Twist: Sit upright on your chair, feet flat on the floor. Inhale to stretch the spine, then exhale as you slowly twist to one side, with one hand on the chair's back and the other on the opposite thigh. Maintain a relaxed shoulder position and a long spine. Hold a few breaths before returning to the centre and repeating on the opposite side.

4. Neck Stretches: Sit tall in your chair and lower your right ear to your right shoulder, feeling a stretch along the left side of your neck. Hold for a few breaths, and then switch sides. You can also gently swivel your head to glance over one shoulder and feel a stretch on the other side of your neck. Hold for a few breaths, then repeat on the opposite side.

Incorporating Gentle Stretching into Daily Life
Gentle stretching in chair yoga is appealing since it is accessible and adaptable. Seniors can incorporate these stretches into their daily routine, whether when they wake up in the morning, during breaks throughout the day, or as part of a bedtime relaxation ritual. When it comes to building flexibility, consistency is essential, so try to perform gentle stretching daily to reap the full advantages over time.

Stretching should be approached with mindfulness and awareness, paying attention to your body's signals and respecting its bounds. Never force a stretch or push through pain, as this might cause harm. Instead, go for a soft, comfortable stretch that lets you breathe deeply and relax into the pose.

Improves strength and balance.

Maintaining muscle strength and balance is critical for seniors to remain independent and avoid falling. Chair yoga provides a safe and efficient technique to increase strength and balance without putting undue strain on the body. Seniors can strengthen their muscles and improve their general stability by doing a variety of chair yoga poses that target different muscle areas.

1.2 Effectiveness of Relaxation Techniques

In today's fast-paced world, stress has become an almost ubiquitous aspect of daily life, especially for seniors dealing with health issues, caregiving responsibilities, or other life obstacles. Fortunately, chair yoga provides a sanctuary of calm by incorporating various relaxation techniques. Let's look at how these strategies can improve seniors' mental and physical health.

Deep Breathing for Stress Relief.

Deep breathing is one of chair yoga's most basic but effective relaxing methods. Seniors can stimulate the body's relaxation response and soothe the nervous system by deliberately slowing down their breath and inhaling and exhaling deeply. Deep breathing reduces cortisol, the stress hormone, while improving oxygen supply to the brain, which promotes clarity and focus.

During chair yoga practice, elders are advised to concentrate on the experience of the breath as it enters and exits the body. They may picture breathing calm and serenity while exhaling tension and worry. Seniors who practice breath awareness can achieve a profound sense of inner serenity and resilience, even when facing adversities.

Guided imagery for relaxation and healing.

Another effective relaxing technique used in chair yoga is guided visualization. Seniors can transport themselves to peaceful, ideal places using visualization and imagination, making them feel protected, supported, and at ease. Guided imagery scripts may take seniors through natural sceneries such as a quiet beach or a peaceful forest, allowing them to immerse themselves in their surroundings' sights, sounds, and sensations.

Guided imagery can be especially effective for seniors suffering from chronic pain, anxiety, or other health difficulties. Seniors can lessen pain perception and increase relaxation throughout their bodies by shifting their focus away from discomfort and toward good, healing imagery. With frequent practice, guided imagery can become an effective tool for stress management and overall well-being.

Mindfulness Meditation for Present-Moment Awareness.
Mindfulness meditation is a key component of many chair yoga practices, providing seniors with an effective technique to improve present-moment mindfulness and inner calm. Seniors who practice mindfulness meditation learn to notice their thoughts, feelings, and sensations without judgment, which helps them create a deeper sense of clarity and calm.

In chair yoga, mindfulness meditation frequently focuses on a specific topic of attention, such as the breath, a mantra, or a bodily sensation. Seniors are asked to bring their entire consciousness to the present moment, detecting any thoughts or distractions that may occur and gently returning their attention to the chosen topic of focus. Over time, mindfulness meditation helps to quiet the mind, reduce stress, and induce a deep state of relaxation.

The Holistic Advantages of Relaxation Techniques
The relaxation techniques used in chair yoga have far-reaching advantages beyond stress reduction. These strategies promote a sense of peace and well-being, which benefits seniors' mental and emotional health and improves their overall quality of life. According to studies, frequent relaxation practices can help seniors manage symptoms of anxiety, sadness, and insomnia, as well as improve cognitive function and immunity.

Furthermore, relaxing techniques significantly impact physical health, affecting everything from blood pressure and heart rate to digestion and immune function. Seniors who reduce stress and promote relaxation may benefit from various health markers, leading to a higher sense of energy and resilience.

Supports weight loss and management.

Let's look at how chair yoga can help elders lose weight. While chair yoga may not burn as many calories as other strenuous exercise types, it has numerous distinct benefits that can help with weight loss and control.

Promotes Mindful Eating.

One of the most important aspects of successful weight loss and management is mindful eating, which is paying attention to hunger cues, eating carefully, and appreciating each meal. Chair yoga enables elders to exercise awareness daily, including mealtimes.

Seniors who practice mindfulness meditation and deep breathing can gain a better understanding of their bodies' hunger and fullness signals. They learn to distinguish between physical and emotional hunger, making it simpler to make informed, healthy eating choices. Seniors who sit down and savour their meals can completely enjoy the flavours and textures of their food, resulting in increased satisfaction and less overeating.

Enhances metabolic function.

While chair yoga may not be as physically taxing as other types of exercise, it can have metabolic benefits that can aid in weight loss and control. Chair yoga involves gentle motions and stretches that enhance circulation and increase blood flow throughout the body. Increased circulation can promote metabolism, resulting in more efficient calorie burning and energy expenditure.

Furthermore, chair yoga postures that work large muscular groups like the legs, arms, and core can help you gain lean muscle mass. Muscle tissue is more metabolically active than fat tissue; having more muscle means burning more calories at rest. Seniors who incorporate strength-building poses into their practice can improve muscle mass and speed up their metabolism, making achieving and maintaining a healthy weight easier.

Reduces Stress and Emotional Eating.

Stress is a common source of emotional eating, and many people rely on food for comfort or distraction.

Chair yoga, which focuses on relaxation techniques like deep breathing and mindfulness meditation, can help seniors cope with stress and minimize emotional eating behaviours.

Seniors can escape the stress and emotional eating cycle by practising chair yoga to cultivate a sense of tranquillity and inner peace. They learn to listen to their bodies and respond to their needs with compassion and self-care rather than using food as a coping technique. As a result, people may find it simpler to make healthy food choices and stick to a well-balanced diet that helps them lose weight.

Improves sleep quality.
Quality sleep is critical for weight reduction and overall health because it controls the hormones influencing hunger and metabolism. Unfortunately, many seniors suffer from sleep disorders like insomnia or restless leg syndrome, which can disrupt the body's natural rhythms and lead to weight gain.

Chair yoga promotes relaxation and stress reduction, making it an effective natural treatment for sleep problems. The gentle exercises and relaxation techniques used in chair yoga can help seniors relax before bedtime, preparing their bodies and minds for a good night's sleep. Seniors who incorporate chair yoga into their nighttime routine may notice increased sleep quality and duration, leading to better overall health and weight management.

Improving Metabolism with Chair Yoga

Elaborate on this Subheading: Improving Metabolism with Chair Yoga

Regular physical activity, such as chair yoga, can assist seniors to improve their metabolism and maintain a healthy weight. Chair yoga positions with moderate motions and fluid sequences can improve circulation and metabolism, allowing seniors to burn calories more efficiently.

1.3 Mindful Eating and Physical Awareness

In today's environment, where food is available, and many people eat mindlessly, mindful eating provides a refreshing alternative. Chair yoga improves physical health and enables seniors to connect more deeply with their bodies and food. Let's look at how the principles of mindful eating and body awareness promoted by chair yoga can help seniors maintain good eating habits and manage their weight.

Understanding Mindful Eating.
At its foundation, mindful eating brings conscious awareness to the entire eating experience, from selecting what to eat to the sensations felt while eating and the emotions that develop afterwards. Rather than eating automatically or in response to external cues such as stress or boredom, mindful eaters listen to their bodies hunger and fullness signals and approach food with curiosity and nonjudgment.

During chair yoga, seniors are encouraged to apply the mindfulness techniques they learn on the mat to their eating habits. They learn to slow down and enjoy each bite, focusing on their food's flavour, texture, and aroma. Seniors who eat deliberately can completely enjoy the nourishment and pleasure that food brings, resulting in increased satisfaction and less overeating.

Cultivating Body Awareness

In addition to mindful eating, chair yoga develops body awareness, or the ability to tune into and comprehend bodily sensations and signals. Chair yoga poses, and relaxation techniques help seniors learn to listen to their bodies and respond to their needs with care and compassion.

Body awareness is especially important for healthy eating and weight control in seniors because it allows them to notice hunger and fullness cues and differentiate between physical and emotional hunger. Seniors can prevent mindless eating by listening to their bodies cues and making more mindful, healthier meal choices that meet their needs.

Practice Mindful Eating Techniques

Seniors can incorporate mindful eating practices into everyday routines to promote healthy eating and weight management. Here are a few strategies inspired by chair yoga:

1. Mindful Meal Preparation: Set aside time to plan and prepare meals consciously, paying attention to the ingredients and cooking process. Engage all of your senses while you cut, season, and cook, taking in the food's sights, scents, and textures.

2. Mindful Eating Rituals: Establish mealtime rituals to improve mindfulness and enjoyment. Before you eat, carefully set the table, light a candle, or say a thanksgiving prayer. Take a moment of stillness to centre yourself before taking the first mouthful.

3. Savor Each Bite: Take your time chewing each bite of food, allowing yourself to enjoy the flavours and sensations. Place your utensils between bites, breathe, and check in with your body.

4. Listen to Your Body: Stay aware of your body's hunger and fullness cues throughout the meal. Eat until you're content, not stuffed, and listen to your body's signals to quit eating when you're no longer hungry.

5. Practice Gratitude: Develop an attitude of gratitude for the nourishment and enjoyment that food brings. Take a moment to thank everyone who helped make the lunch possible.

Benefits of Mindful Eating and Body Awareness
Seniors can benefit from mindful eating and body awareness in ways that go beyond weight management. This includes:

- Enhanced digestion and nutrition absorption.
- Reduced stress and anxiety about food
- Increased satisfaction and enjoyment of meals
- Increased understanding of food choices and desires.
- Better self-regulation and impulsive control with food

Finally, mindful eating and body awareness allow seniors to gain control of their health and well-being, resulting in a more balanced and harmonious relationship with food and their bodies.

Chapter 2. Understanding Weight Loss and Aging

In this chapter, we will look at the relationship between weight loss and the ageing process. As we age, our bodies undergo various changes that affect our metabolism, body composition, and capacity to lose weight. But don't worry; we can navigate these changes with the correct knowledge and tactics and meet our weight loss objectives.

2.1 Aging Metabolism: Understanding the Slowdown.

Metabolism is frequently compared to the engine that powers our bodies, transforming the food and beverages we ingest into the energy required to perform our everyday activities. It is a complex process involving several biochemical reactions within our cells. However, as we age, this once-efficient engine begins to sputter and slow down, resulting in a drop in metabolic rate.

This metabolic slowdown might be due to various variables, including hormonal changes, muscle loss, and decreased physical activity. As a result, our bodies become less efficient at burning calories, making it easier to gain excess weight, particularly in the middle.

But do not worry because there are ways we may use to combat this natural drop in metabolism. Regular exercise is one of the most effective techniques since it has been found to enhance metabolic rate and calorie burn during and after physical activity. Activities that include strength training and high-intensity interval training (HIIT) are especially useful for increasing metabolism.

Strength training, such as weightlifting or resistance exercises, aids in developing and maintaining lean muscle mass. Muscle tissue is more metabolically active than fat tissue; thus, having more muscle can result in a greater resting metabolic rate, which means you burn more calories even when you are not exercising. Furthermore, HIIT workouts, which consist of short bursts of intense activity followed by rest or lower-intensity exercise, have been found to enhance metabolic rate and calorie burning for hours after the session.

Now, chair yoga comes into the picture. While chair yoga may not be as intense as typical strength training or HIIT workouts, it provides unique advantages that can contribute to a faster metabolism. The moderate movements and poses in chair yoga activate and engage numerous muscle groups, increasing muscle strength and endurance. Furthermore, emphasizing deep breathing and mindfulness in chair yoga might help reduce stress, which may support a healthier metabolism.

So, if you're concerned about your metabolism slowing as you get older, realize that you can keep that metabolic engine working smoothly. Regular exercise, especially activities such as chair yoga, can help reverse the effects of ageing on your metabolism and keep you at a healthy weight for years to come.

2.2 Body Composition Changes: Understanding Sarcopenia.

As we age, our bodies experience a variety of alterations, one of which is a shift in body composition. This shift is most obvious with the development of Sarcopenia, a disorder marked by the gradual loss of muscular mass and strength, which is frequently accompanied by a rise in body fat percentage.

Sarcopenia can have a far-reaching impact on our general health and well-being. It not only causes decreases in physical strength and functional capacity, but it also plays an important role in the development of chronic illnesses such as osteoporosis, insulin resistance, and metabolic syndrome.

So why does Sarcopenia occur? Hormonal changes, decreased physical activity, and poor food choices are all contributing reasons. As we age, our bodies become less efficient at manufacturing protein, which is the building block of muscle tissue, resulting in a steady loss in muscle mass. Furthermore, lifestyle variables such as sedentary behaviour and insufficient protein consumption might worsen muscle loss over time.

But don't worry; there's a lot we can do to counteract Sarcopenia and keep our valuable muscle mass. Enter strength training, fitness's superhero. Strength training entails executing activities that put your muscles up against resistance, such as lifting weights, using resistance bands, or, you guessed it, chair yoga.

Chair yoga may not appear to be a conventional strength training routine, but be aware of its mild demeanor. Chair yoga poses and motions are intended to engage and build muscle groups throughout the body, including the legs, arms, core, and back. By including regular chair yoga practice into your regimen, you can effectively counteract muscle loss while maintaining or increasing muscle mass over time.

However, the benefits of strength training go beyond muscle maintenance. Building and maintaining lean muscle tissue will increase your strength, balance, and general functional fitness. This means you'll be better able to carry groceries, climb stairs, and play with your grandchildren.

So, if you're concerned about how your body composition changes as you age, realize that you can defy the odds and keep a strong, healthy body. By including strength training techniques such as chair yoga, you may prevent Sarcopenia, enhance your metabolism, and maintain a vibrant, active lifestyle well into your golden years.

2.3 Hormonal Changes: Getting Around the Hormonal Roller Coaster.

Hormones are the silent orchestrators of our bodies' symphony, regulating everything from mood to metabolism. As we age, these hormonal maestros can endure severe plot twists, resulting in variations that affect our weight and general health. Menopause is a natural transition that signals the end of menstruation and causes a cascade of hormonal changes.

During menopause, estrogen levels decrease, causing changes in body composition and fat distribution. Women may notice an increase in abdominal fat, also known as visceral fat, which has been related to an increased risk of chronic conditions, including heart disease and diabetes. Furthermore, variations in estrogen levels can alter how our bodies respond to food, making it easier to acquire weight and more difficult to lose.

But don't worry; while we can't stop the passage of time or reverse the hormonal changes accompanying menopause, we can encourage hormone balance and appropriate weight control. One of the most effective ways is to focus on lifestyle factors that promote hormonal health.

First and foremost, emphasize nutrition. A well-balanced diet rich in whole foods, such as fruits and vegetables, lean meats, and healthy fats, provides your body with the resources it requires to support hormone production and regulation. Certain nutrients, such as omega-3 fatty acids and antioxidants, have been proven to promote hormonal balance and reduce inflammation, potentially alleviating menopausal symptoms.

In addition to nutrition, frequent exercise is essential for hormone balance and weight management. Physical activity regulates hormone levels, reduces stress, and improves mood, benefiting hormonal health. Try cardiovascular exercise, strength training, and flexibility exercises like chair yoga to maintain your body strong, fit, and resilient.

Stress management is another critical component in maintaining hormonal health. Chronic stress can disturb hormone balance and lead to weight gain, particularly in the middle. Stress-reduction techniques like deep breathing, meditation, and mindfulness can assist in relaxing the nervous system and produce a sense of balance and well-being.

Last but not least, prioritize sleep. Quality sleep is critical for hormone control, metabolism, and overall well-being. Aim for 7-9 hours of restful sleep per night, and stick to a consistent sleep pattern to support your body's natural circadian cycles.

So, while hormone changes are unavoidable in the ageing process, there's no reason to fear. Focusing on nutrition, exercise, stress management, and sleep can help you maintain hormone balance, encourage healthy weight management, and negotiate the hormonal roller coaster with grace and grit. Remember that you can support your body's natural rhythms and accept the changes with each stage of life.

2. 4 Mindset Matters: Developing a Positive Outlook.

The role of thinking in weight loss and overall well-being cannot be emphasized. Our thoughts, beliefs, and attitudes toward ourselves and our bodies impact our behaviors and, ultimately, our success in pursuing a better lifestyle. As we age, it becomes more important to cultivate a positive mindset that allows us to overcome obstacles, set realistic objectives, and appreciate our accomplishments along the way.

First and foremost, let's tackle the elephant in the room: negative self-talk. It's easy to fall into the trap of self-criticism and doubt, especially when dealing with every weight reduction journey's unavoidable setbacks and challenges. But here's the thing: that inner critic serves no one, least of all you. Cultivate self-compassion and gentleness instead of criticizing oneself for perceived flaws or mistakes.

Accept the motto of progress, not perfection. Understand that setbacks are a normal part of the process and provide opportunities for growth and learning. Rather than obsessing over past mistakes or what might have been, concentrate on the current moment and the modest actions you can take daily to get closer to your goals.

Setting attainable goals is another essential component of developing a good mentality. While it is important to dream large and aspire high, unreasonable expectations can lead to disappointment and frustration. Break down your ambitions into smaller, more doable steps, and celebrate each accomplishment. Whether fitting into a favourite pair of pants or completing a chair yoga practice without getting winded, every accomplishment, no matter how minor, is worth celebrating.

Also, surround yourself with positivity and encouragement. Look for friends, family, or online communities that share your goals and may provide support, accountability, and inspiration. Remember that you are not alone; we are all on this path together, and there is strength in unity.

Finally, be grateful. Take a minute each day to reflect on what you're thankful for: the love and support of family and friends, the beauty of nature, or your body's power and resilience. Cultivating a grateful attitude can help you adjust your perspective and focus on the gifts in your life rather than perceived flaws.

Chapter 3: Getting Started with Chair Yoga

In this chapter, we're diving into the wonderful world of chair yoga and exploring how you can get started on your journey to improved health and well-being. Whether you're a seasoned yogi or brand new to the practice, chair yoga offers a gentle yet effective way to reap the benefits of yoga, regardless of age or fitness level.

3.1 Understanding Chair Yoga

First things first, let's talk about what exactly chair yoga is. Chair yoga is a modified form of traditional yoga practiced sitting on a chair or using a chair for support. It incorporates gentle stretches, breathwork, and mindfulness techniques to improve flexibility, strength, and relaxation. The beauty of chair yoga is that it can be adapted to suit individuals with various physical limitations or mobility issues, making it accessible to virtually everyone.

Choosing the Right Chair

Before diving into your chair yoga practice, choosing the right chair is essential. Look for a sturdy, stable chair with a flat seat and backrest. Stay away from chairs with wheels or arms that restrict movement. Ideally, you want a chair that allows you to sit comfortably with your feet flat on the floor and your knees at a 90-degree angle. For added comfort and support, you can place a non-slip mat or cushion on the seat.

Setting the Scene

Next, create a peaceful and inviting space for your chair yoga practice. Find a quiet area free from distractions where you can fully focus on your practice. Consider dimming the lights, playing soft music, or lighting a candle to enhance the ambiance and promote relaxation. Ensure you have enough room to move comfortably around your chair without obstructions.

Warm-Up Exercises

Before diving into the yoga poses:
1. Take a few moments to warm up your body and prepare for practice.
2. Start by sitting tall in your chair with your feet flat on the floor and your hands resting on your thighs. Your eyes should be closed, and take several deep breaths, inhaling through your nose and exhaling through your mouth.
3. Allow your breath to flow naturally, filling your lungs with oxygen and releasing tension or stress with each exhale.

Next, gently roll your shoulders up, back, and down in a smooth, circular motion, loosening any tension in your neck and shoulders. Rotate your wrists and ankles, flexing and extending each joint to improve circulation and mobility. Finally, stretch your arms overhead, reaching the sky as you lengthen through your spine. Take a few deep breaths here, feeling the stretch in your side body and upper back.

Closing Meditation
To conclude your chair yoga practice:
1. Take a few moments to sit quietly and meditate.
2. Close your eyes and bring your awareness to your breath, noticing the rise and fall of your chest with each inhale and exhale.
3. Allow your breath to anchor you in the present moment, letting go of any thoughts or distractions that may arise.
4. Take a few moments to express gratitude for yourself and your body, honoring the time you've dedicated to your practice.

Chapter 4: Chair Yoga Poses for Weight Loss

In this chapter, we'll look at chair yoga poses specifically intended to help people lose weight. Chair yoga is a gentle yet effective way to improve strength, flexibility, and metabolism, all of which are necessary for a successful weight loss journey. So take a chair, settle into a comfortable position, and join us as we explore a variety of positions to help you on your path to a healthier, happier you. 20 chair yoga positions intended specifically for seniors to help with weight loss, along with their benefits:

1. Tadasana (Seated Mountain Pose)

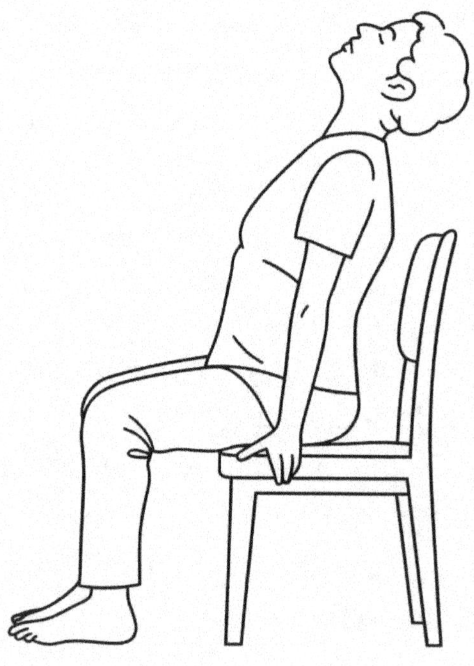

- Sit tall on your chair, feet flat on the floor, and hands resting on your thighs.
- Extend your spine, retract your shoulders, and lift your chest.

- Close your eyes and take a few deep breaths, concentrating on your sit bones and reaching toward the summit of your head.

Benefits
Seated Mountain Pose enhances posture, strengthens core muscles, and promotes a sense of grounding and stability. It also encourages bodily awareness and attention.

2. Seated Forward Bend (Paschimottanasana)

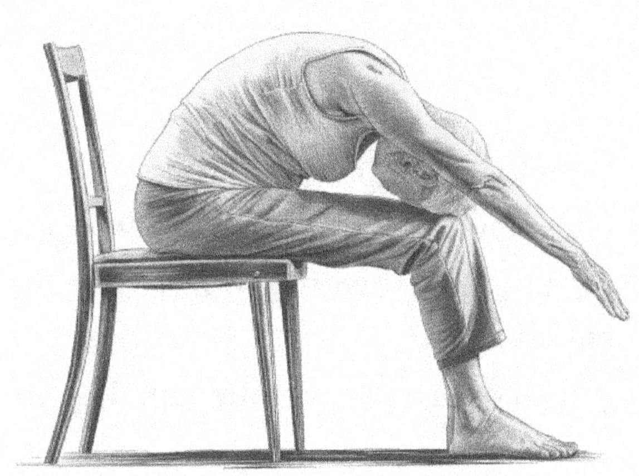

- Sit on the edge of your chair, feet flat on the floor, hip-width apart.
- Inhale deeply to stretch your spine, then exhale while tilting forward from your hips and folding your torso over your thighs.
- Let your arms hang down to the floor or hold the edges of your chair.

Benefits
The seated forward bend stretches the hamstrings, calves, and lower back, improving flexibility and reducing tension. It also improves digestion and promotes calm.

3: The Seated Cat-Cow Stretch

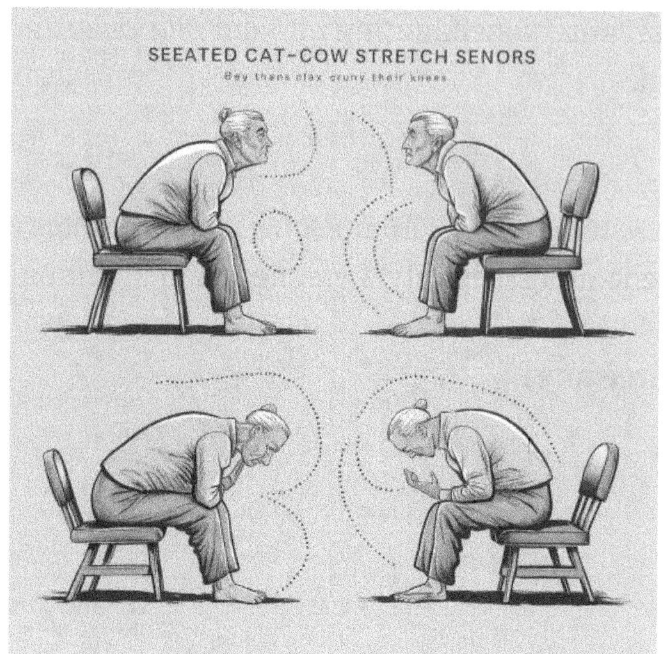

- Sit tall on your chair, feet flat on the floor, and hands resting on your knees.
- Inhale while arching your back, raising your chest, and looking up (Cow Pose).
- Exhale while curving your back, tucking your chin toward your chest, and bringing your belly button toward your spine (cat stance).
- Alternate between Cat and Cow Pose, moving softly and gently with each breath.

Benefits

The Seated Cat-Cow Stretch improves spinal flexibility, stretches back muscles, and encourages relaxation and stress relief. It promotes both circulation and digestion.

4. The Seated Warrior Pose (Virabhadrasana)

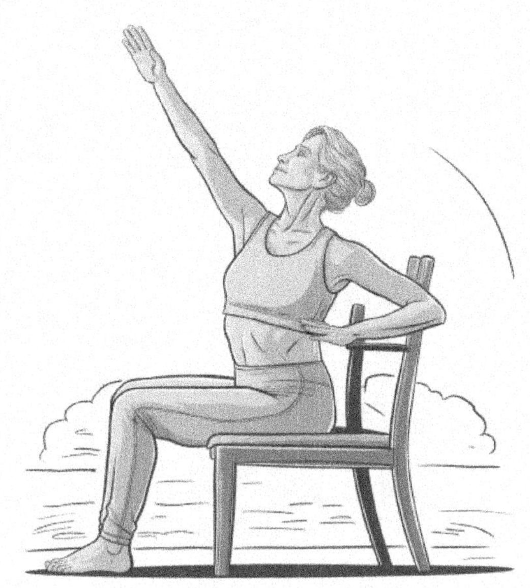

- Sit tall in your chair, feet hip-width apart and hands resting on your thighs.
- Inhale deeply and extend your arms to the heavens.
- Engage your core muscles and press down on your sit bones to feel a stretch in your side body.

Benefits
Seated Warrior Pose strengthens the arms, shoulders, and core muscles, which improves balance and stability. It also energizes the body and boosts confidence and empowerment.

5. Seated Twist (Ardha Matsyendrasana)

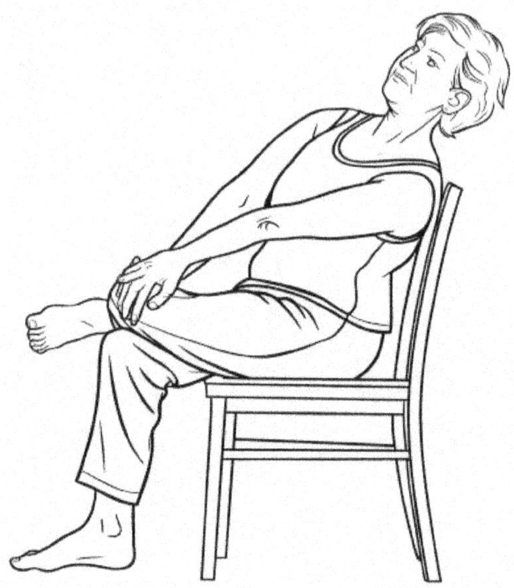

- Sit tall on your chair, feet flat on the floor, and hands resting on your thighs.
- Inhale deeply to lengthen your spine, exhale, and twist your torso to the right.
- Place your left hand on the outside of your right leg and your right hand against the chair's back.

Benefits

The Seated Twist stretches the spine, shoulders, and hips, promoting spinal mobility and digestion. It also detoxifies the body, reducing bloating and soreness.

6. Seated side stretch (Parsva Sukhasana)

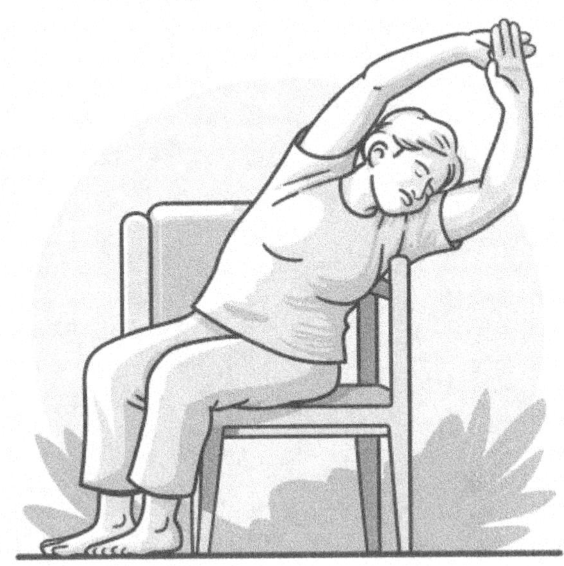

Sit comfortably in your chair; your feet should be flat on the floor. Inhale, then raise your arms overhead, interlocking your fingers and raising your palms toward the ceiling.

- Exhale and progressively lean to one side, resulting in a deep stretch along the opposite side of your body.

Benefits
The Seated Side Stretch lengthens the side body, stretches the intercostal muscles, and improves lateral flexibility. It also stimulates digestion and increases circulation.

7. Seated Eagle Arms (Garudasana Arms)

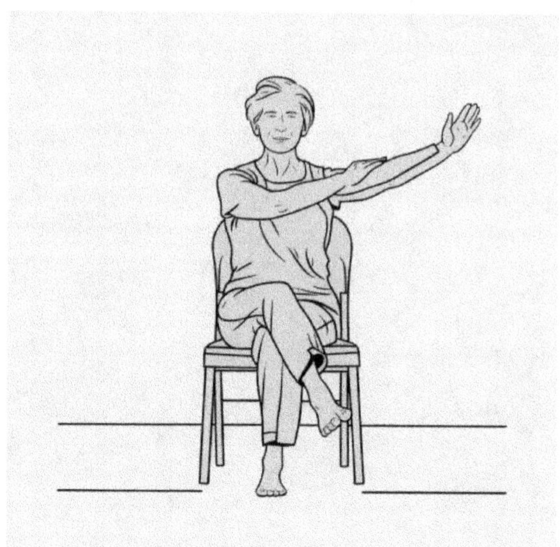

- Sit upright on your chair, feet flat on the floor and arms relaxed at your sides. Inhale, then extend your arms out to the sides, shoulder height.
- Exhale, then cross your right arm over your left, bending your elbows and maybe wrapping your forearms together.

Benefits
Seated Eagle Arms stretch the shoulders and upper back, resulting in better posture and less strain. It also improves focus and concentration while relaxing the mind and reducing stress.

8. Seated High Lunge (Utthita Ashwa Sanchalanasana)

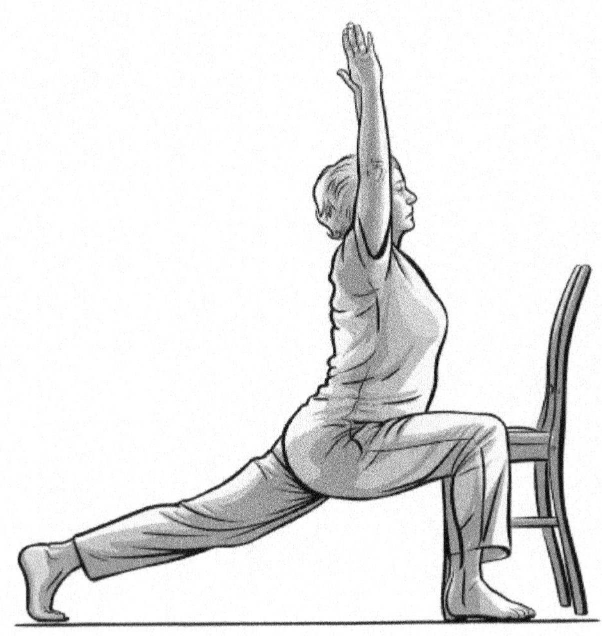

- Sit on the front edge of your chair, feet flat on the ground.
- Extend your right leg behind you, with toes tucked under and heel lifted.
- Lift your chest and raise your arms overhead, using your core and pressing down with your left foot.

Benefits

Seated High Lunge exercises develop the legs, glutes, and core muscles, resulting in better balance and stability. It also extends the hip flexors and quadriceps, reducing stiffness and pain.

9. Seated boat pose (Navasana)

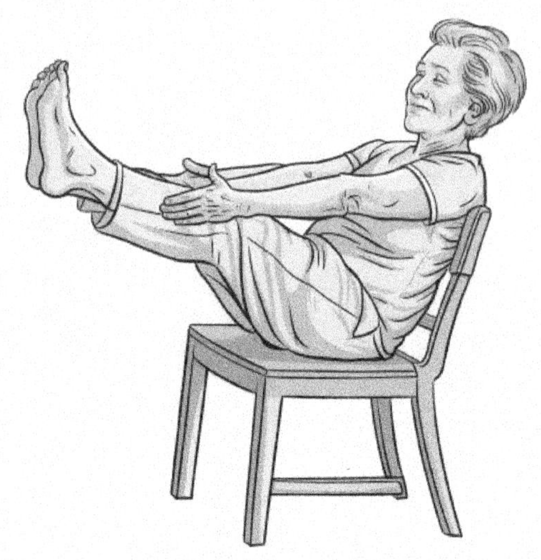

- Sit on the front edge of your chair, feet flat on the ground.
- Lean back slightly and raise your feet off the floor, bringing your shins parallel to the ground.
- Extend your arms forward beside your legs, palms facing inwards.

Benefits
Seated Boat Pose strengthens the core muscles, especially the abdominals and hip flexors, improving balance and stability. It also stimulates the digestive tract and promotes cleaning.

10. The Seated Goddess Pose (Utkata Konasana)

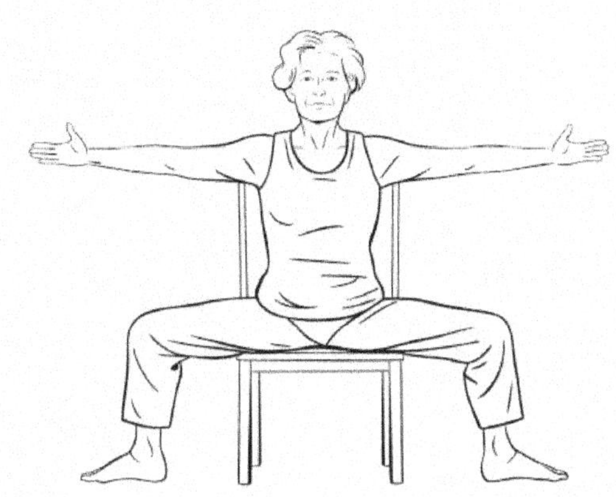

- Sit tall on your chair, feet flat on the floor, and knees bent.
- Inhale, then extend your arms to the sides at shoulder height, palms facing forward.
- Exhale and bend your knees into a wide-legged stance.

Benefits
Seated Goddess Pose strengthens the legs, glutes, and inner thighs, improving lower-body strength and stability. It also stretches the hips and pelvis, improving flexibility and movement.

11. Seated Extended Triangle Pose (Utthita Trikonasana)

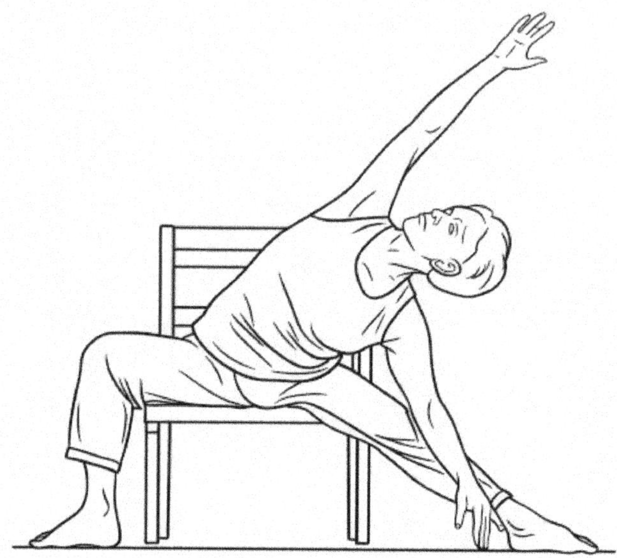

- Sit at the front edge of your chair, legs spread wide.
- Inhale, extend your arms to the sides, shoulder height.
- Exhale and extend your right hand toward your right foot, bending at the waist and raising your left hand to the ceiling.

Benefits

The Seated Extended Triangle Pose stretches the hamstrings, inner thighs, and side body, which improves flexibility and spinal alignment. It also improves digestion and cleaning.

12. Seated Cow Face Pose (Gomukhasana Arms)

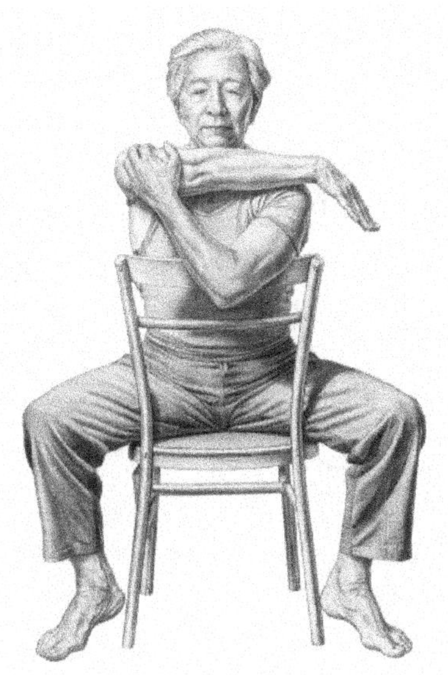

- Sit tall on your chair; your feet should be flat on the floor.
- Cross your right arm over your left, bending your elbows and perhaps wrapping your forearms together.

Benefits
Seated Cow Face Pose stretches the shoulders, arms, and upper back, improving posture and reducing tension. It also enhances focus and concentration, calming the mind and relieving stress.

13. Seated butterfly pose (Baddha Konasana)

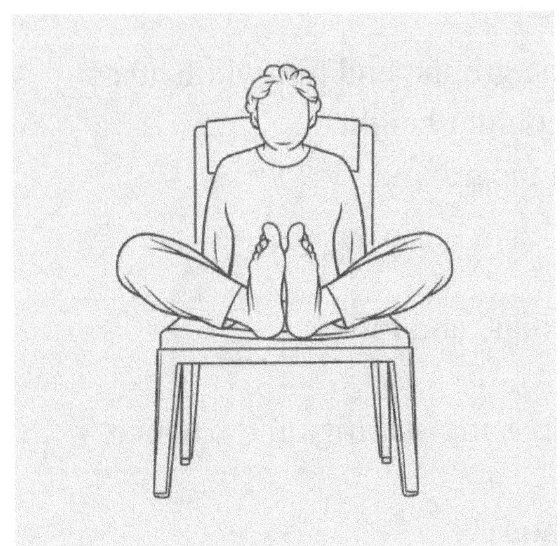

- Sit tall on your chair, feet flat on the floor, and knees bent.

- Bring your foot soles together and allow your knees to drop to the sides.

Benefits

The seated butterfly pose stretches the inner thighs, groins, and hips, increasing flexibility and mobility. It also stimulates stomach organs and promotes relaxation.

14. Seated Garland Pose (Malasana)

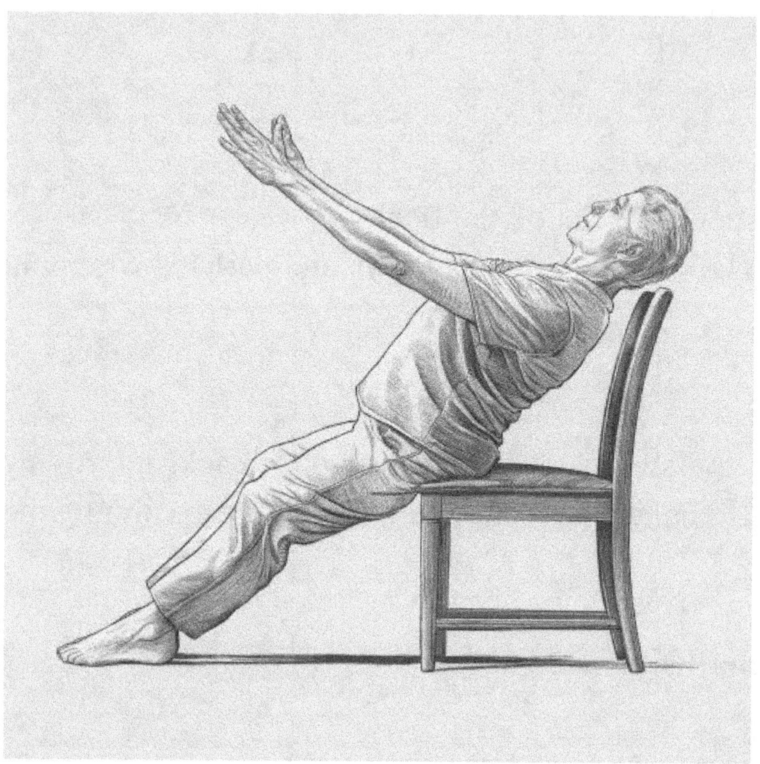

- Sit at the front edge of your chair, feet flat on the ground and hip-width apart.
- Inhale and raise your arms out to the sides at shoulder height.
- Exhale, bend your knees and bring your hips to the ground.

Benefits:

 The seated garland posture stretches the hips, groins, and lower
I am back, improving flexibility and mobility.
It also strengthens the legs and core muscles, increasing stability and balance.

15. Seated Half Moon Pose (Ardha Chandrasana)

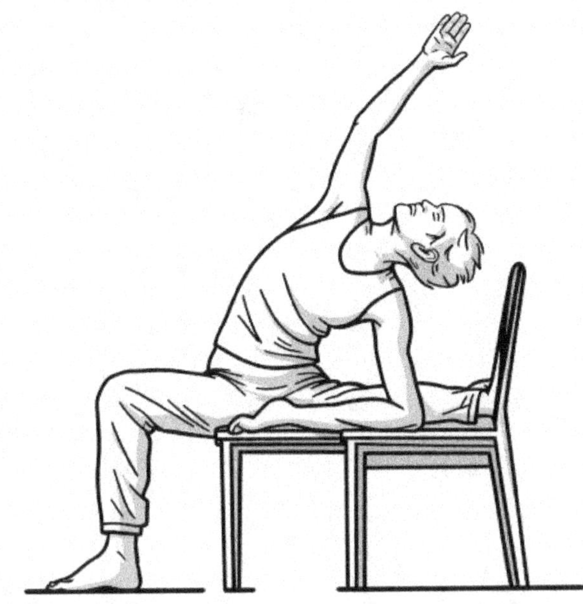

- Sit on the front edge of your chair, feet flat on the ground.
- Inhale, then raise your arms overhead, interlocking your fingers and raising your palms toward the ceiling.
- Exhale and progressively lean to one side, resulting in a deep stretch along the opposite side of your body.

Benefits
The seated half-moon posture stretches the side body, widens the ribcage, and improves spinal flexibility. It also stimulates digestion and increases circulation.

16. Seated tree pose (Vrksasana)

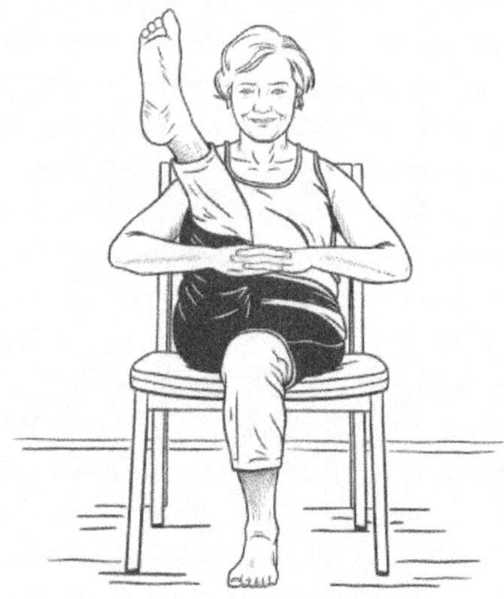

- Sit down tall on your chair; your feet should be flat on the floor.
- Lift your right foot off the ground and place the sole against the inner left thigh or calf.
- Press your right foot into your left leg while contracting your core muscles.

Benefits: The seated tree posture improves balance, concentration, and stability. It also strengthens the legs and core muscles, improving posture and alignment.

17. Seated Staff Pose (Dandasana).

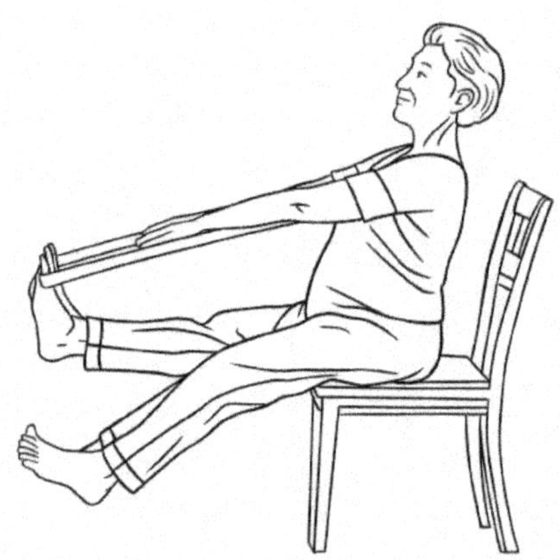

- Sit on the front edge of your chair, legs straight in front of you and feet flexed.
- Place your hands on the armrests of your chair or your thighs.

Benefits

Seated Staff Pose strengthens the quadriceps, hamstrings, and core muscles, improving posture and balance. It also stretches the spine and promotes good spinal alignment.

18. Seated Extended Hand-to-Big Toe Pose (Utthita Padangusthasana)

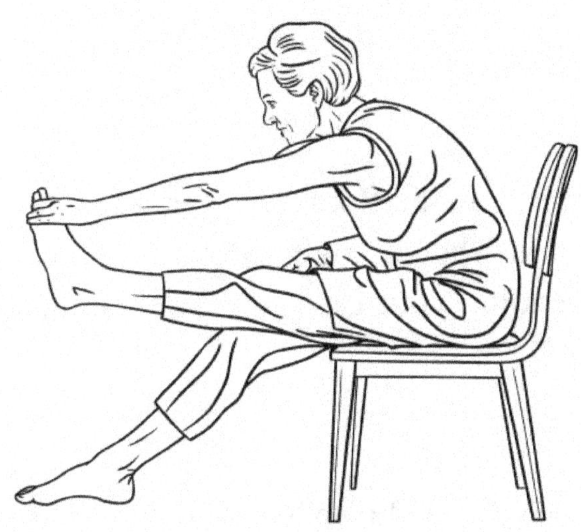

- Sit on the front edge of your chair, legs straight in front of you.
- Inhale and lift your right leg off the floor, stretching it straight ahead.
- Reach your right hand toward your right foot, gripping the big toe if feasible.

Benefits

The seated extended hand-to-big-toe pose stretches the hamstrings, calves, and hip flexors, improving flexibility and mobility. It also strengthens the core muscles, increasing balance and stability.

19. Seated Warrior II Pose (Virabhadrasana II)

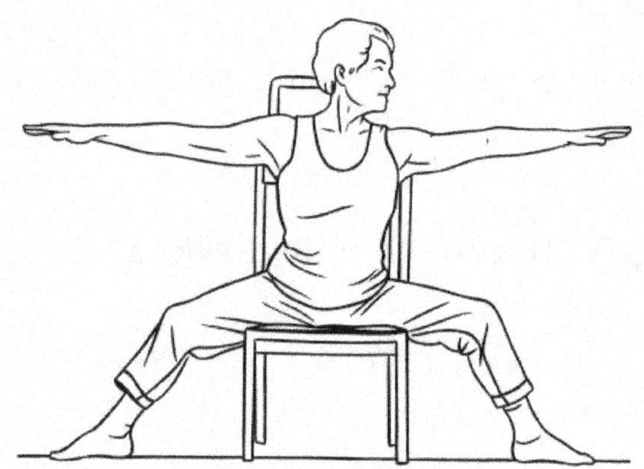

- Sit toward the front edge of your chair, feet flat on the floor, legs spread wide.
- Inhale, extend your arms to the sides to shoulder height, palms down.
- Exhale and shift your torso to the right, bending your right knee and connecting with your right ankle.

Benefits
Seated Warrior II Pose strengthens the legs, opens the hips and chest, and improves balance and stability. It also enhances focus and concentration, calming the mind and reducing tension.

20. Seated Wide-Legged Forward Bend (Upavistha Konasana)

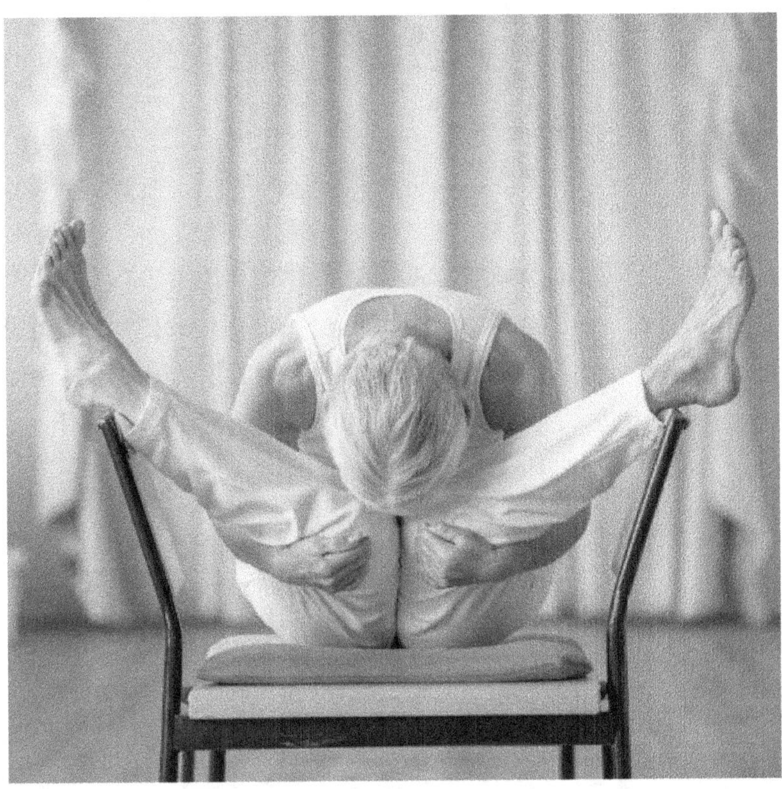

- Sit at the front edge of your chair, extending your legs out in a V shape. Inhale deeply to stretch your spine, then exhale while bending forward from your hips and folding your torso over your thighs.

Benefits
Sit wide-legged forward. Bend stretches the inner thighs, hamstrings, and lower back, increasing flexibility and reducing tension. It also stimulates stomach organs and promotes relaxation.

Incorporating these chair yoga techniques throughout your daily practice will help elders lose weight. Remember to practice consciously, listening to your body and understanding its limitations. You'll experience greater strength, flexibility, and overall well-being with consistent practice and dedication.

Chapter 5: Chair Yoga Routines for Seniors

This chapter will examine various chair yoga practices that benefit seniors' health and wellbeing. These gentle yet effective routines employ seated poses, breathing exercises, and mindfulness techniques to improve flexibility, strength, balance, and vitality. Whether you are new to chair yoga or an experienced practitioner, these routines include something for everyone, regardless of age or fitness level.

5.1 Why Should Seniors Perform Chair Yoga Routines?

Before we get started, let's discuss why chair yoga is especially beneficial for seniors. Maintaining flexibility, strength, and mobility as we age is vital to our overall health and pleasure of life. On the other hand, traditional forms of exercise may be difficult or inaccessible to seniors due to joint pain, decreased mobility, or balance issues. Chair yoga is a safe and accessible alternative that allows seniors to reap the benefits of yoga without having to lie on the floor or strain their bodies.

1. Safety and Accessibility: Chair yoga is designed to be safe and accessible for people of all ages and fitness levels, including seniors. Unlike traditional yoga practices, which may require seniors to lie on the floor, chair yoga allows them to perform modest stretches and motions while sitting in a solid and comfortable chair. This reduces the likelihood of falls or injuries when attempting more challenging postures on the mat.

2. Joint Health: Many elders experience joint discomfort or stiffness, making typical exercise difficult or impossible. Chair yoga is a low-impact strategy for enhancing joint health that gently moves the joints through their whole range of motion. The chair's supportive design allows elders to move without putting undue stress on their joints, reducing discomfort and improving flexibility over time.

3. Improved Flexibility: As people age, their flexibility decreases, resulting in less movement and a higher risk of injury. Chair yoga programs comprise gentle stretching movements designed to improve muscle flexibility and range of motion. Regular practice can help seniors maintain or increase their flexibility, making daily tasks easier and decreasing the likelihood of falls or accidents.

4. Muscle Building: Maintaining muscle strength is essential for seniors' balance, stability, and overall functional independence. Chair yoga programs contain strength-building movements that target specific muscle groups such as the core, legs, and arms. These exercises improve muscle tone and strength without heavy weights or equipment, making them ideal for seniors looking to stay strong and active as they age.

5. Balance and Stability: As we age, balance and stability become more crucial for preventing falls and maintaining independence. Chair yoga programs include poses and exercises that demand balance and coordination, which helps seniors improve their strength and reduce their risk of falling. The chair offers a safe environment for older adults to practice balancing skills, gradually increasing confidence and stability.

6. Mind-Body Connection: Chair yoga is more than just physical exercise; it also incorporates elements of mindfulness and relaxation. Deep breathing, meditation, and guided relaxation are helpful for seniors to reduce stress, improve mental clarity, and boost their sense of wellbeing. These activities can be especially beneficial for seniors who are dealing with chronic pain, anxiety, or other stress-related issues.

Overall, chair yoga routines offer a comprehensive approach to senior health by addressing wellness's physical, mental, and emotional aspects. Chair yoga allows seniors to take control of their health and enjoy a healthier lifestyle well into their golden years by offering a safe, accessible, and effective form of exercise.

5.2 Set Up Your Chair Yoga Space

Before starting your chair yoga practice, you should create a comfortable and appealing environment to fully concentrate on your training. Choose a quiet, distraction-free location with enough space to move around your chair easily. Dim the lights, play soft music, or light a candle to create a calm mood. Keep supports like a yoga strap, bolster, or blanket nearby to help with your practice.

Creating a comfortable atmosphere for your chair yoga practice is essential for a satisfying and effective session. Here's why it's important and how to set up your chair yoga area:

1. Reduce Distractions: Choosing a quiet, distraction-free setting allows you to immerse yourself fully in your practice without interruption. Turn off external noise sources like the television, phones, and conversations to create a relaxing and concentrated environment.

2. Enhance Ambiance: By reducing the lights or setting them to a soft, warm glow, you can create a tranquil ambiance that encourages relaxation and alertness. Soft lighting calms the senses and fosters calmness, making concentrating on your breathing and movement simpler throughout practice.

3. Use Gentle Music or Sounds: Placing calm music or natural sounds in the background will enhance the atmosphere of your chair yoga room. Choose calming songs or ambient noises such as running water or birdsong to create a peaceful environment that supports your practice and allows you to unwind.

4. Set the Mood with Scent: Consider using aromatherapy to boost the atmosphere in your chair yoga setting. Lighting a scented candle or using essential oils in a diffuser can fill the space with pleasant scents such as lavender, chamomile, or eucalyptus, known for their calming and stress-reducing properties.

5. Prepare Your Props: Keeping yoga props such as a yoga strap, bolster, or blanket handy will aid you in practice and provide support when needed. A yoga strap can aid in deepening stretches and increasing flexibility, while a bolster or blanket can provide additional support during relaxation poses. These materials allow you to modify positions and adjust based on your requirements and preferences.

6. Create a Sacred Space: Make your chair yoga practice a sacred ritual by setting aside special time and space in your daily schedule. Choose a tranquil part of your home or a room where you can practice uninterrupted and adorn it with motivating things like candles, crystals, or inspirational quotes. Creating a sacred space honors your practice while instilling reverence and focus.

Making your chair yoga practice environment more comfortable and inviting will improve your entire experience and help you get more out of your sessions. Setting up your chair yoga environment by removing distractions, boosting the ambiance, or including props in your practice allows you to fully immerse yourself in the present moment and connect with your body, breath, and inner quiet.

5.3 Breathing Warm-Up Routine

Let's start with a slow breathing warm-up to relax your mind and ready your body for exercise. Sit tall in your chair, feet level with the floor and hands resting on your thighs. Close your eyes and breathe deeply in through your nose and mouth. As you breathe, imagine inflating your belly like a balloon on the inhale and gradually drawing your navel closer to your spine on the exhale. Continue to breathe deeply and regularly, letting each breath relax your mind and body.

The **Breathing Warm-Up Routine** is an essential chair yoga practice for focusing the mind, connecting with the breath, and preparing the body for movement. Here's a more detailed explanation of its importance and how to accomplish it:

1. Mindfulness: Creating a sense of mental focus and presence is vital before beginning any physical activity. The breathing warm-up technique starts with sitting straight in your chair, closing your eyes, and focusing inward. By reducing external distractions and focusing inward, you create an environment conducive to mindfulness and self-awareness, establishing the framework for a more attentive and deliberate practice.

2. Connecting with the Breath: The breath is a powerful tool for relaxing, reducing stress, and cultivating a sense of calm. During the breathing warm-up routine, inhale deeply through your nose and exhale through your mouth. This deliberate breathing technique oxygenates the body, boosts circulation, and activates the parasympathetic nervous system, causing a relaxation response. Paying attention to the rhythm and quality of your breath allows you to stay in the present moment and anchor your consciousness there.

3. Balloon Breathing: Imagine filling your abdomen with air like a balloon on the inhale and slowly dragging your navel towards your spine on the exhale to deepen and control your breathing. As you inhale deeply, imagine your belly expanding like a balloon filled with air, letting the breath circulate throughout your abdomen. On the exhale, gently contract your abdominal muscles to bring the navel closer to the spine, exhaling fully and completely. This diaphragmatic breathing technique stimulates the lungs, enhances oxygen exchange, and aids in relaxation and stress reduction.

4. Mind-Body Connection: The breathing warm-up technique strengthens the connection between the mind and body, allowing you to synchronize your breath with your movements and achieve inner peace and balance. Continue to breathe deeply and rhythmically, allowing each breath to take you deeper into calm and awareness. Consider how the quality of your breath affects your body and mind, and then allow yourself to relax into the natural rhythm of your breathing.
The breathing warm-up exercise is a gentle yet effective way to begin your chair yoga practice, preparing you for a concentrated and embodied experience. By concentrating on the mind, connecting with the breath, and focusing on the present moment, you lay the framework for a practice that benefits the body, mind, and soul. So, take a few seconds to practice this simple yet effective breathing warm-up technique and allow yourself to be transformed by mindful breathing.

5.4 Gentle Stretching and Mobility.

This program includes modest stretching and mobility exercises to improve joint flexibility and range of motion. Sit tall in your chair, feet level with the floor and hands resting on your thighs. To reduce neck and shoulder stiffness, gently move your shoulders up, back, and down in a smooth, circular motion. Then, raise your right arm overhead and reach to the left side of the room, feeling a stretch down your right side. Hold for a few breaths, then switch over to the other side. Next, interlace your fingers behind your back and gently squeeze your palms together to form an opening in your chest and shoulders. Hold for a few breaths, then release and repeat. Finally, bring your right ear to your right shoulder, which will extend the left side of your neck. Hold for a few breaths, then switch sides. Continue these stretches while taking deep breaths and listening to your body.

The Chair Yoga Routines

Routine 1: Moderate Stretching and Mobility

Moderate Stretching and Mobility aims to improve flexibility and joint mobility through moderate and accessible movements. The following is a complete breakdown of its components and their significance.

1. Improving Flexibility and Range of Motion: Flexibility and mobility are important aspects of overall physical health, especially as we age. This regimen targets these areas by incorporating gentle stretching exercises that lengthen muscles and enhance joint range of motion. Seniors who do these stretches regularly can improve their flexibility, reduce stiffness, and maintain a wider range of motion, contributing to greater mobility and functional independence.

2. Improving Joint Health: Many seniors suffer from joint stiffness and discomfort, limiting their ability to do everyday duties and leading to a worse quality of life. The modest stretching movements in this program help to lubricate the joints, reduce stress, and relieve stiffness, resulting in better joint health and comfort. Regularly doing these stretches can help seniors enhance the health and longevity of their joints, allowing them to move more freely and comfortably.

3. Releasing Tension: Muscle tension and stiffness can lead to discomfort and restricted movement. The gentle stretching in this practice helps release stress in important body parts, including the neck, shoulders, chest, and spine. Seniors can feel more at ease and comfortable in their bodies by consciously relaxing tight muscles and lowering areas of tension, which promotes relaxation and stress reduction.

4. Improving Posture: Poor posture is common among seniors and can lead to musculoskeletal issues, including back pain, neck strain, and reduced mobility. This routine's stretches are intended to open up the chest and shoulders, counteracting the effects of slouching and rounded shoulders. Seniors can improve their posture and alignment to relieve muscle and joint strain, enhance breathing and circulation, and boost comfort and wellbeing.

5. Mind-Body Connection: As with all chair yoga routines, this one emphasizes connecting with your breath and listening to your body. Breathing deeply and purposefully as you progress through each stretch can help you feel more conscious and present in the moment. Paying attention to your body's sensations and understanding your limitations allows you to practice safely and effectively while not pushing yourself too hard.

Moderate Stretching and Mobility exercise offers elders a gentle but effective method for increasing flexibility, improving joint health, and promoting relaxation. Seniors who implement these stretches into their daily routine will feel more comfortable, mobile, and vital, allowing them to enjoy life to the fullest.

Routine 2: Strength and Stability

This program focuses on strengthening and stabilizing the muscles, notably in the core, legs, and arms. Sit tall in your chair, feet level on the floor, hands resting on your thighs. Begin by contracting your core muscles and raising one foot, stretching it out before you. Hold for a few breaths before lowering and switching sides. Next, place your hands on your chair's armrests and push down, using your chest and arm muscles. Hold for a few breaths before releasing and repeating. Finally, extend your arms to the sides and rotate your palms to face forward, activating the shoulder muscles. Hold for a few breaths before releasing and repeating. Remember to keep your posture and alignment correct throughout the exercise and to breathe deeply with each movement.

The Chair Yoga Routine 2: Strength and Stability targets major muscle groups while increasing overall strength and stability. Here's a more in-depth description of its components and significance:

1. Core Strength: Core strength is critical for maintaining stability and good posture, especially as we age. This practice includes workouts that strengthen and support the spine by engaging core muscles such as the abdominals and lower back. Seniors activate their core muscles to maintain balance and control by elevating one foot off the floor while sitting erect in the chair. This strengthens the core muscles, improves posture, and lowers the chance of falls and accidents.

2. Leg Strength: Strong legs are essential for movement, balance, and functional independence. The practice includes workouts to strengthen the leg muscles, such as the quadriceps, hamstrings, and calves. Lifting one foot off the floor and extending it in front of the body works the leg muscles, increasing strength and stability. This activity helps elders keep strong and steady legs, simplifying walking, climbing stairs, and standing up from a seated position.

3. Arm Strength: Upper body strength is required for daily tasks such as reaching, lifting, and carrying goods. The practice includes workouts to develop arm muscles such as the chest, shoulders, and arms. Seniors can strengthen and stabilize their upper bodies by pushing down on the chair's arms with their hands. This exercise promotes arm strength, good posture, and general functional fitness.

4. Shoulder Stability: Strong and stable shoulders are necessary for good posture and avoiding shoulder problems. The practice includes workouts to strengthen the shoulder muscles, specifically the deltoids and rotator cuff. Seniors can strengthen their shoulder muscles and improve joint stability by stretching their arms to the sides and twisting their palms to face forward. This exercise improves shoulder strength, mobility, and resilience, which reduces the likelihood of shoulder pain or injury.

5. Maintaining Good Posture: Proper posture is essential for maintaining stability, balance, and general spinal health. The activity asks elders to sit erect in their chairs, feet level on the floor, and hands resting on their thighs. This helps to align the spine, activate the core muscles, and promote good posture and alignment. Seniors can increase the efficiency of their exercises while lowering their risk of strain or injury by keeping proper posture throughout the regimen.

The Strength and Stability program provides seniors a targeted and effective strategy to increase strength, improve stability, and promote overall functional fitness. Seniors who incorporate these exercises into their normal regimen will benefit from increased strength, stability, and confidence in their everyday activities, improving their quality of life and encouraging healthy aging.

Routine 3: Rest and Stress Relief.

This program emphasizes relaxation and stress alleviation, which helps settle the mind and promotes peace and wellbeing. Sit tall in your chair, feet level on the floor, hands resting on your thighs. Begin by closing your eyes and taking a few deep breaths through your nose and out through your mouth. As you breathe, imagine a wave of tranquility rolling over your body, beginning at the top of your head and descending to your toes. Continue to breathe deeply and regularly, allowing each breath to increase your level of relaxation. Next, focus your attention on your body and observe any places of tension or discomfort. As you exhale, envision releasing the tension and letting your body soften and relax. Continue breathing and relaxing for many minutes, allowing yourself to unwind and completely release stress or tension. When you're ready, slowly open your eyes and return your focus to the present now, feeling refreshed and invigorated.

Relaxation and Stress Relief is a relaxing practice for seniors that aims to help them unwind, relieve tension, and build a deep sense of wellbeing. Let's look at the components of this procedure in greater detail:

1. Deep Breathing: The regimen starts with techniques that help calm the mind and encourage relaxation. Seniors engage the parasympathetic nerve system by inhaling deeply through the nose and gently expelling through the mouth, causing the body to relax. This deep breathing technique reduces stress, lowers blood pressure, and promotes peace and contentment.

2. Visualization: Visualization is highly effective for generating relaxation and alleviation. In this technique, seniors are urged to imagine a wave of relaxation washing over their body, beginning at the top of the head and descending to the toes. This visualization helps to focus the mind, relieve tension, and produce a sensation of calm and spaciousness in the body. Seniors can improve their sense of peace and wellbeing by imagining themselves relaxed.

3. Body Scan: The body scan technique entails bringing awareness to various body areas and identifying any points of tension or discomfort. With each breath, seniors are advised to visualize releasing tension and allowing the body to soften and relax. This focused awareness of the body aids in identifying and releasing accumulated stress, resulting in physical relaxation and mental clarity.

4. Mindful Relaxation: Throughout the program, seniors are encouraged to practice mindful relaxation by paying attention to their breath, thoughts, and feelings without judgment. Seniors who observe their experiences with curiosity and compassion can strengthen their connection to the present moment and let go of worries or concerns. This mindfulness practice reduces stress, improves mood, and promotes overall wellbeing.

5. Gentle Movement: While this program emphasizes relaxation and stress alleviation, gentle movement can be included to help promote relaxation and release tension in the body. Simple movements like modest neck rolls, shoulder shrugs, and wrist circles can relieve stress and increase circulation, improving the relaxing experience.

6. Closing and Integration: The practice closes with a delicate return to the present moment, allowing seniors to return their attention to their surroundings gradually. Seniors can incorporate the benefits of relaxation into their daily lives by gently opening their eyes and taking a few seconds to reorient themselves, leaving them feeling refreshed, invigorated, and ready to tackle the rest of their day with renewed energy and vitality.

Overall, the Relaxation and Stress Relief routine provides:

- Seniors with a quiet and revitalizing exercise to relieve stress, c.
- Calming Mind, and.
- Cultivating a sense of relaxation and wellbeing. Seniors

Incorporating these activities into their daily routines can increase their resilience to stress, improve their general quality of life, and promote a stronger sense of peace and harmony.

Chapter 6: Incorporating Chair Yoga into Daily Life

In this chapter, we'll look at practical methods to incorporate chair yoga into your everyday life so you can consistently reap the benefits of this mild yet effective practice. Let's plunge in!

6.1 Practical methods to incorporate chair yoga

1. Start Small and Build Consistency:

Including chair yoga in your regular practice does not have to be difficult. Begin by putting aside a few minutes daily for a quick chair yoga session. Whether in the morning to get your day started, during a work break, or in the evening to decompress before bed, please choose a time that works best for you and stick to it. Consistency is crucial, so practice chair yoga daily, even for a few minutes.

Starting small and gradually increasing Consistency is a fundamental element for implementing chair yoga into your everyday routine. Let's dig deeper into why this strategy is useful and how you may use it:

1. Overcoming Overwhelm: Many fear adding another activity to their already packed calendars. Start simple, such as with a few minutes of chair yoga daily, to make the practice feel more doable and less daunting. This can help remove any reservations you may have about getting started.

2. Creating a Sense of Accomplishment: Starting with simple, attainable goals allows you to experience immediate wins and a feeling of accomplishment. Even a little chair yoga session can leave you feeling renewed, motivated, and proud of yourself for prioritizing your health. This positive reinforcement motivates you to keep the habit and raise the duration or intensity of your practice over time.

3. Consistency is the key to success when forming new habits: Committing to a daily chair yoga practice, even if only for a few minutes, generates momentum and positive momentum. Over time, Consistency helps to establish the habit and smoothly integrate chair yoga into your everyday routine.

4. Finding the correct Time: Choosing the proper time to practice chair yoga is critical for maintaining Consistency. Please choose the most convenient time, whether first thing in the morning to establish a positive tone for the day, during a lunch break to recharge and refocus, or in the evening to unwind and relax before bed. Consistency is simpler when your practice becomes ingrained in your everyday routine.

6. 2. Make It A Habit

Make chair yoga a habit and include it in your everyday routine. Please select a specific signal or trigger to remind you to practice, such as setting an alarm on your phone, placing a sticky note on your desk, or associating it with another regular ritual, such as brushing your teeth or preparing your morning coffee. By constantly matching chair yoga with a specific cue, you may reinforce the habit and make it simpler to maintain over time.

Making chair yoga a habit is key for incorporating it into your daily routine. Let's look into how you may make chair yoga a habit:

1. Identify a Cue or Trigger: A cue or trigger is a precise prompt that signifies the beginning of your chair yoga session. It might be anything you associate with practicing yoga, such as setting an alarm on your phone for a specific time of day, putting a sticky note on your desk or refrigerator, or connecting it to another regular practice, such as brushing your teeth, making your morning coffee, or taking a lunch break. Choose a cue consistent with your current habit and easy to recall.

2. Consistency is key: Regularly pairing chair yoga with your selected cue is essential for reinforcing the habit. Please commit to practicing chair yoga whenever your cue comes, whether daily, weekly, or at set times throughout the day. Consistency strengthens the relationship between the cue and the behavior, making it easier to recall and perform over time.

3. Start Small: As previously said, starting small is critical to developing a new habit. Begin by committing to a few minutes of chair yoga every time your cue appears. Beginning with a modest time makes the habit seem less intimidating and more attainable. As the habit becomes ingrained, you can progressively intensify your practice.

4. Create a Routine: Creating a consistent routine around your chair yoga practice might help to reinforce the habit. Choose a consistent time and location for practice each day, whether before breakfast, during your lunch break, or in the evening before bed. By including chair yoga into your daily routine, you establish a structure that reinforces the habit and makes it simpler to sustain over time.

5. Track Your Progress: Keeping track of your progress will help you stay accountable and inspired as you attempt to develop the habit of chair yoga. Keep a notebook or use a habit-tracking app to document each practice session and any thoughts or observations about how you felt before and after. Seeing your improvement over time can be extremely motivating and help you stay committed to the practice.

6. Be Patient and Persistent: Developing a new habit takes time and effort, so be patient with yourself as you begin your chair yoga practice. Keep going even if you miss a day or make a mistake. Instead, concentrate on getting back on track and renewing your dedication to the habit. With practice and determination, chair yoga can become a natural and joyful part of your daily routine, resulting in better health, wellbeing, and quality of life.

6. 3. Be flexible and Adaptable.

Life can be unpredictable, and finding time for a full-chair yoga practice may be difficult. That is okay! Be adaptable and open to changing your practice to accommodate your schedule. If you only have a few minutes to spare, try simple stretches and breathing exercises. Remember that even a brief practice is preferable to none, and every bit helps improve your health and wellbeing.

Flexibility and adaptability are essential when implementing chair yoga into your routine. Here's a more in-depth look at why this strategy is important and how you can properly use it:

1. Managing Life's Challenges: Life can be hectic and unexpected, and finding time for a complete chair yoga practice on certain days may seem impossible. Instead of being disheartened or giving up entirely, being flexible allows you to tailor your practice to your current situation. Whether you have a hectic schedule, unforeseen commitments, or limited time, flexibility will enable you to stick to your self-care and wellbeing goals despite life's difficulties.

2. Embracing Imperfection: Regarding chair yoga, perfection is not the goal. Instead of trying for an idealized notion of what your practice should be, embrace imperfection and focus on doing your best with the time and resources you have. Being adaptable allows you to let go of fixed expectations and approach your practice with curiosity and acceptance.

3. Making the Most of Limited Time: Even if you only have a few minutes, a reduced chair yoga practice can still provide benefits. By focusing on a few easy stretches or breathing exercises, you can reap yoga's physical, mental, and emotional advantages in a shorter period. Remember that every bit of movement and mindfulness contributes to better health and wellbeing, so don't underestimate the power of a brief practice.

4. Prioritizing Self-Care: Being adaptable with your chair yoga practice entails prioritizing self-care and realizing the significance of looking after yourself, even when life gets hectic. By devoting even a modest amount of time each day to self-care techniques such as chair yoga, you demonstrate a dedication to your health and wellbeing. This dedication is required to preserve balance and resilience in life's obstacles.

5. Adjusting to Changing Needs: As your life circumstances change, so will your capacity to practice chair yoga similarly. Being adaptable helps you tailor your practice to your changing requirements and preferences. Whether you have physical restrictions, health concerns, or changes in your daily schedule, being adaptive allows you to continue reaping the advantages of chair yoga while adjusting any adjustments that may occur.

6. 4. Incorporate Chair Yoga into Daily Activities

You do not need to set aside time for chair yoga; it may be smoothly integrated into your everyday routine. Practice deep breathing while waiting in line at the grocery store, sitting stretches while watching TV, or include mindfulness practices in your daily walks. By incorporating chair yoga into your daily routine, you may optimize its advantages without adding extra time to your schedule.

Integrating chair yoga into everyday activities is a simple and efficient method to make it a routine. Here's an in-depth look at why and how you may incorporate chair yoga into your regular activities:

1. Maximizing Efficiency: In today's fast-paced world, finding time for extracurricular activities such as chair yoga might be tough. Integrating chair yoga into your daily duties allows you to increase efficiency by mixing yoga practice with chores you perform regularly. This strategy eliminates the need to set aside specific time for yoga, making it simpler to maintain Consistency and prioritize self-care during a hectic schedule.

2. Making the Most of Downtime: Many daily activities require downtime or waiting, such as standing in line, attending appointments, or commuting. Instead of wasting this time, could you make the most of it by doing chair yoga? Whether deep breathing while waiting in line at the grocery store, seated stretches while watching TV, or practicing mindfulness on your daily walks, incorporating chair yoga into these activities allows you to maximize your free time while promoting physical and mental wellbeing.

3. Improving Mind-Body Connection: Incorporating chair yoga into your daily routine fosters a stronger mind-body connection by bringing your attention to your body and breathing throughout the day. Incorporating yoga practices such as deep breathing, stretching, and mindfulness into your daily activities promotes a sense of presence and mindfulness that permeates all aspects of your life. This increased awareness can assist in reducing stress, improving concentration, and boosting general wellbeing.

4. Tailoring Yoga to Your Lifestyle: Incorporating chair yoga into your regular activities may personalize your practice to your needs and interests. Instead of following a traditional yoga timetable or framework, you can tailor your training to your current needs. This individualized approach guarantees that yoga remains accessible and pleasurable, increasing the likelihood that you will persist with it over time.

5. Promoting Consistency: Consistency is essential for obtaining the benefits of chair yoga. Integrating yoga into your regular activities provides built-in reminders and opportunities for practice throughout the day. This continuous exposure to yoga reinforces the habit and makes it a natural part of your routine, increasing overall Consistency and commitment to your wellness goals.

6. 5. Customize Your Practice

Make chair yoga your own by tailoring it to your requirements and interests. Try different positions, stretches, and breathing methods to see what feels best for your body. Please don't hesitate to change positions or add props to make them more accessible or comfortable. Chair yoga is flexible to all fitness levels and abilities, so don't be afraid to customize your practice to meet your specific needs.

Customizing your chair yoga practice is critical to making it pleasurable, accessible, and successful for your specific requirements and preferences. Here's a deeper look at why personalization is crucial and how you may adjust your practice to meet your particular needs:

1. Personalization: Everyone is unique, so what works for one person may not work for another. Customizing your chair yoga practice allows you to personalize it to your specific goals, limits, and preferences. Whether you are looking to improve flexibility, relieve pain, reduce stress, or improve your general wellbeing, tailoring your practice allows you to focus on the important areas.

2. Accessibility: Chair yoga is adjustable to all fitness levels and abilities, making it available to almost anybody. By tailoring your practice, you can adapt poses and methods to whatever physical restrictions or obstacles you may face. For example, if you have restricted movement or flexibility, you can utilize props like blocks or straps to help you practice and make poses easier. Customizing your practice allows you to engage fully and comfortably, regardless of your fitness level or physical condition.

3. Comfort and Safety: Customizing your chair yoga practice allows you to be more comfortable and safe while practicing. By altering poses or utilizing props as needed, you can avoid discomfort or strain and lower your risk of injury. For example, suppose you feel uncomfortable in specific postures or have a history of joint pain. In that case, you can modify the pose or use props to support your body and relieve pressure on sensitive regions. Prioritizing comfort and safety enables you to practice with confidence and peace of mind.

4. Exploration and Variety: By customizing your chair yoga practice, you can experiment with various poses, stretches, and breathing methods, keeping your practice fresh and fascinating. Experiment with sequences, variants, and combinations to determine what works best for your body and mind. Do not be scared to be innovative and try new things. Variety not only keeps you from becoming bored, it also guarantees that you're targeting different muscle groups and areas of your health for a more complete workout.

5. Empowerment and Ownership: Customizing your chair yoga practice to meet your requirements and preferences allows you to take control of your health and wellbeing. Rather than taking a one-size-fits-all approach, you actively participate in your wellness journey, choosing decisions consistent with your values and objectives. This sensation of empowerment promotes a stronger connection to your practice, increasing its effectiveness and impact.

Celebrate your progress.
Finally, remember to enjoy your accomplishments along the road. Whether improving your flexibility, feeling more peaceful and centered, or simply incorporating chair yoga into your daily routine, every step forward is worth celebrating. Recognize your efforts and triumphs, and be proud of yourself for putting your health and wellbeing first through chair yoga.

Including chair yoga in your daily routine improves physical, mental, and emotional health. By starting small, making it a habit, being flexible and adaptable, incorporating it into your everyday activities, tailoring your practice, keeping encouraged and inspired, and celebrating your progress, you can make chair yoga a long-term and meaningful part of your lifestyle.
Celebrating your progress is an important part of your chair yoga experience. Here's why and how you can make the most of it:

1. Recognizing Achievements: Celebrating your development encourages you to acknowledge and appreciate your accomplishments. Whether you've observed gains in your flexibility, strength, balance, or overall wellbeing, recognizing these achievements reinforces the benefits of your chair yoga practice and encourages you to keep going.

2. Celebrating your achievement: increases your confidence and motivation, allowing you to stay devoted to your chair yoga practice. Recognizing the positive improvements you've seen reminds you of your abilities and perseverance, motivating you to overcome obstacles and continue on your wellness journey.

3. Celebrating your progress: fosters thankfulness and happiness, helping you to focus on the wonderful things in your life. Appreciating the benefits of chair yoga and the good changes it has brought about helps to create an abundant mindset, which leads to increased general contentment and wellbeing.

4. Creating Momentum: Celebrating your progress generates momentum and propels you onward in your chair yoga adventure. As you celebrate your accomplishments, you create momentum that will carry you through challenges and failures, encouraging you to keep working toward your goals.

5. Deepening Self-Awareness: Celebrating your accomplishment stimulates self-reflection and self-awareness, helping you to obtain insights into your strengths, weaknesses, and places for improvement. Recognizing your progress and achievements enables you to better understand yourself and your talents, allowing you to make educated decisions and manage problems confidently.

Finally, praising your accomplishment increases resilience and resilience, allowing you to recover from failures and setbacks. Focusing on your accomplishments and the positive parts of your chair yoga practice fosters a resilient mindset, enabling you to endure adversity and emerge stronger and more resilient than before.

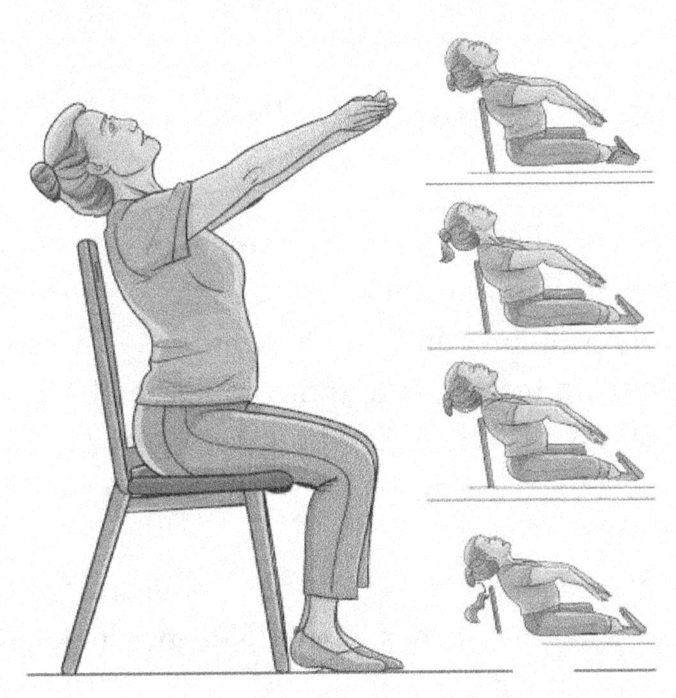

Chapter 7: Nutritional Considerations for Weight Loss

In this chapter, we'll look at nutrition's critical role in obtaining and maintaining a healthy weight. While chair yoga is a fantastic way to improve physical fitness and overall well-being, it's important to supplement your practice with a healthy diet. Let's look at some crucial nutritional concerns for your weight loss quest.

7.1. Eat a Balanced Diet.

A balanced and healthy diet is the cornerstone of any successful weight loss program. Incorporate various nutritious foods into your meals, including fruits, vegetables, lean meats, whole grains, and healthy fats. These nutrient-dense meals supply critical vitamins, minerals, and antioxidants, making you feel satiated and invigorated. Avoid overly processed foods, sugary snacks, and excessive amounts of saturated fats and refined carbs, as they can all lead to weight gain and bad health effects.

A balanced diet is the foundation of every successful weight loss strategy, and it's critical to understand what that means. Here's a deeper look at the significance of a balanced diet and how to attain it:

1. Variety of Whole Foods: Try to integrate a variety of whole foods into your meals. These include fruits, vegetables, lean proteins, grains, and healthy fats. Each of these food groups contains critical nutrients for overall health and well-being. Fruits and vegetables are high in vitamins, minerals, and antioxidants, whereas lean proteins aid in tissue construction and repair, and whole grains include fibre that promotes digestive health. Avocados, almonds, and olive oil are healthy fats for brain function and hormone management.

2. Nutrient Density: Choose foods that are nutrient dense, which means they contain a high concentration of nutrients per calorie. Nutrient-dense foods not only nourish your body, but they also keep you satiated for longer, lowering your chances of overeating. Nutrient-dense foods include leafy greens, strawberries, salmon, quinoa, and almonds.

3. Avoid Highly Processed Foods: Limit your intake of highly processed foods, which are frequently heavy in added sugars, harmful fats, and artificial ingredients. These foods have minimal nutritional value and can lead to weight gain and a variety of health issues, such as heart disease, diabetes, and inflammation. Instead, opt for whole, less processed foods whenever possible.

4. Limit Sugary Snacks: Sugary snacks and desserts can add extra calories to your diet while delivering minimal nourishment. While it is acceptable to indulge in indulgences occasionally, strive to restrict your intake of sugary foods and beverages regularly. When you need a sweet treat, choose healthier options such as fresh fruit, Greek yogurt with honey, or dark chocolate with almonds.

5. Limit Saturated Fats and Refined carbs: While fats and carbs are vital macronutrients, not all sources are equal. Limit your consumption of saturated fats, which can be found in animal products such as red meat and full-fat dairy, as well as processed foods like fried dishes and pastries. Instead, choose healthier fats like nuts, seeds, avocados, and olive oil. Similarly, select nutritious grains like brown rice, quinoa, and oats over refined carbohydrates such as white bread, pasta, and sugary cereals.

7. 2. Portion Control.

Portion control is critical for regulating calorie intake and encouraging weight loss. Pay attention to serving sizes and avoid large meals, especially when eating out or with prepared foods. Smaller dishes, bowls, and utensils will allow you to control portion sizes and prevent overeating. Furthermore, mindful eating, which involves savoring each bite, eating deliberately, and paying attention to hunger and fullness cues, might help you avoid mindless snacking and excessive calorie consumption.

Portion control is essential to weight management and can significantly impact your ability to meet weight loss objectives. Let's look at why portion control is important and how to implement it efficiently:

1. Managing Calorie Intake: Portion control helps limit your calories, which is critical for weight loss. You can avoid overeating by controlling your meals and consuming fewer calories than your body requires. This is especially crucial when dining out or eating packaged foods, as portion sizes in restaurants and pre-prepared meals are frequently greater than needed.

2. Preventing Overeating: Even if the food is nutritious, overeating might occur due to large servings. Paying attention to serving sizes and selecting proper portions will help you avoid ingesting excess calories and retain greater control over your hunger. Using smaller plates, bowls, and utensils might visually deceive your brain into believing you're eating more than you are, allowing you to feel fuller with smaller portions.

3. Mindful Eating: Mindful eating is another excellent approach to portion control. This entails paying special attention to the sensory experience of eating, such as flavor, texture, and aroma. By savoring each bite and eating slowly, you allow your body to register sensations of fullness, lowering the risk of overeating. Listening to your body's hunger and fullness cues can also help you know when to stop eating, keeping you from consuming unneeded calories.

4. Strategies for Success: You may utilize various practical strategies to incorporate portion management into your everyday routine. Begin by learning the normal serving sizes for protein, grains, or veggies. Portion suitable amounts of food using measuring cups, spoons, or a scale, especially if you cook at home. Consider splitting entrée with a buddy or ordering fewer servings from the menu when dining out. And remember that it's fine to leave food on your plate if you're full rather than feeling obligated to eat it.

5. Consistency is vital for portion control: Make it a habit to exercise portion management at all meals and snacks rather than just on occasion. Over time, these little alterations can result in large changes in your calorie consumption and total weight. Be patient with yourself and strive for progress rather than perfection, as mastering portion control is a skill that takes time and practice to develop.

Stay Hydrated.

Drinking enough water promotes general health and can aid in weight loss. Water regulates metabolism, removes toxins, and keeps you feeling full and content. Aim for at least eight glasses of water daily, and try sipping water throughout the day, especially before meals, to help reduce your hunger. Herbal drinks, flavored water, and sparkling water can all be refreshing alternatives to plain water that will keep you hydrated.

Staying hydrated is important to sustaining general health and helping weight loss attempts. Let's go deeper into why hydration is important and how to ensure you're getting enough fluids.

1. Water regulates metabolism: the process by which your body turns food and drink into energy. Staying hydrated ensures your metabolism runs smoothly, helping you burn calories efficiently and aid in weight loss. Dehydration can impede metabolism, making it more difficult to lose excess weight.

2. Toxin Removal: Hydration is crucial for eliminating toxins and waste from your body. Drinking enough water promotes kidney function, allowing kidneys to filter out pollutants and maintain optimal fluid balance properly. Staying hydrated promotes your body's natural detoxification processes, which can help with weight loss and overall wellness.

3. Drinking water can help you regulate your appetite and avoid overeating. Feelings of thirst are often misinterpreted as hunger, resulting in excessive snacking and calorie consumption. Staying hydrated allows you to distinguish between thirst and hunger cues, ensuring you meet your body's demands correctly.

Drinking water before meals will help you feel fuller and lower your chances of overeating.

4. Daily Hydration Goals: Aim for at least eight glasses of water daily, while individual hydration requirements may differ depending on age, gender, activity level, and weather. Keeping a water bottle with you throughout the day can remind you to drink regularly while also allowing you to track your fluid intake. Herbal teas, fruit or herb-infused water, and sparkling water might help you keep hydrated and enjoy it more.

5. Hydration and Physical Activity: Staying hydrated is especially important during activity since you lose fluids through sweat. Drink water before, during, and after physical activity to replace lost fluids and avoid dehydration. Monitoring your urine color can also be a good measure of your hydration level; strive for pale yellow pee, which indicates enough hydration.

6. Consistency is key: Staying hydrated regularly is critical for getting the benefits of optimal hydration. Make it a practice to drink water throughout the day rather than waiting until you are thirsty. Set reminders on your phone or use hydration tracking software to ensure you achieve your daily fluid requirements.

Staying hydrated is essential for good health and can help you lose weight in various ways. You may improve your health and well-being while losing weight by drinking plenty of water, regulating metabolism, flushing out toxins, limiting appetite, and sticking to your hydration routine. Remember, water is your body's best friend, so keep drinking and being hydrated!

7. 3. Focus on Nutrient Density.

When planning your meals and snacks, prioritize foods with high nutritional density, which means they give a considerable amount of nutrients for the calories they contain. Nutrient-dense foods include leafy greens, colourful vegetables, berries, nuts and seeds, lean meats, and whole grains. Eating nutrient-dense meals may fuel your body while promoting weight loss and overall wellness.

The emphasis on nutrient density is important in developing a healthy and effective weight loss plan. Consider why nutrient-dense foods are important and how to incorporate them into your meals and snacks.

1. **Maximizing Nutritional Value:** Nutrient-dense foods contain vitamins, minerals, fiber, and antioxidants, all necessary for overall health and well-being. Unlike empty-calorie foods, which give little nutritional benefit, nutrient-dense foods contain a high concentration of nutrients per calorie. By selecting these meals, you may guarantee that your body receives the nutrients it requires to function properly while consuming fewer calories.

2. **Supporting Weight Loss Goals:** Nutrient-dense foods are essential to a successful weight loss plan since they keep you full and energized while ingesting less calories. Fiber-rich foods, such as leafy greens, vegetables, and whole grains, enhance satiety and appetite control, making it simpler to keep to your calorie targets. Lean proteins like poultry, fish, tofu, and beans promote sensations of fullness while also supporting muscle growth and repair, which is critical for maintaining a balanced metabolism during weight loss.

3. **Promoting Overall Health:** Besides weight loss, eating nutrient-dense foods improves overall health and lowers the risk of chronic diseases, including heart disease, diabetes, and cancer. The vitamins, minerals, and antioxidants present in nutrient-dense foods have a variety of health benefits, including increased immunity, decreased inflammation, and improved cellular function. Incorporating these foods into your diet can improve your general health and longevity.

4. **Practical Tips for Incorporation:** To increase nutrient density in your meals and snacks, include a range of bright fruits and vegetables high in vitamins, minerals, and phytonutrients. Choose whole grains like quinoa, brown rice, and oats over processed grains to boost fiber and nutritional content. To promote muscular health and satiety, incorporate lean proteins such as chicken, turkey, fish,

and eggs and plant-based proteins such as beans and lentils. Snack on nuts, seeds, and Greek yogurt for a filling source of healthy fats and protein.

5. Balanced and Varied Diet: Prioritizing nutrient-dense foods is vital, as is maintaining a balanced and varied diet. Aim to consume a variety of macronutrients (carbohydrates, proteins, and fats) in each meal to ensure that your body gets a full range of nutrients. To avoid overeating, keep portion sizes in check and listen to your body's hunger and fullness cues.

7. 4. Be Mindful of Emotional Eating.

Emotional eating, or eating based on emotions rather than hunger, can sabotage weight loss efforts and lead to harmful eating habits. Pay attention to your emotional eating triggers, such as stress, boredom, or loneliness, and devise coping mechanisms that do not involve food. Mindfulness approaches, such as deep breathing, meditation, or engaging in enjoyable hobbies, can help you manage stress and emotions without turning to food.
Awareness of emotional eating is critical for establishing a healthy relationship with food and achieving weight loss goals. Let's look at why emotional eating happens and how you can use mindfulness to overcome it:

1. Understanding Emotional Eating: Emotional eating is the inclination to use food as a coping method for dealing with feelings like stress, melancholy, boredom, or loneliness rather than eating to satisfy physical hunger. Emotional triggers differ from person to person and may result from past events, societal influences, or taught behaviors. However, turning to food for comfort can result in binge eating, weight gain, and feelings of guilt or shame.

2. Identifying Triggers: Identifying your triggers is the first step toward overcoming emotional eating.

Pay attention to situations, feelings, or events that cause you to seek food when you aren't hungry. Workplace stress, interpersonal issues, boredom in idle periods, and emotions of loneliness or sadness are all common factors. Identifying your triggers allows you to address them and develop healthy coping methods proactively.

3. Developing Coping Strategies: Rather than resorting to food for consolation, consider other coping strategies to manage your emotions properly. Deep breathing, meditation, and progressive muscle relaxation are all mindfulness strategies that can help you stay present and calm during stressful situations. Going for a stroll, practicing a hobby, or spending time with loved ones are all delightful activities that help you avoid emotional eating.

4. Emotional Resilience: Emotional resilience is critical for handling life's obstacles without resorting to food for comfort. Practice self-care behaviours that promote emotional well-being, such as getting adequate sleep, exercising frequently, and putting relaxation first. Create a supporting social network of friends and family members who can offer encouragement, empathy, and understanding at difficult times. By increasing your emotional resilience, you will better deal with stress and emotions healthily.

5. Mindful Eating Practices: Practicing mindful eating can help you become more aware of your body's hunger and fullness cues, lowering the likelihood of emotional eating episodes. Before you eat, check in with yourself to see if you're physically or emotionally hungry. Pay attention to the taste, texture, and satisfaction of each bite, and enjoy the experience of eating without interruptions. Eating thoughtfully allows you to develop a stronger connection with your body and a healthier relationship with food.

6. Seeking Support: If your emotional eating behaviors persist despite your best efforts to change them, hesitate to seek assistance from a healthcare professional or registered dietitian specializing in emotional and disordered eating. They can offer individualized advice, Support, and resources to help you create healthy coping methods and conquer emotional eating difficulties.

7 5. Seek professional Guidance.

If you need help navigating the complexity of nutrition and weight loss independently, consult a licensed dietitian or nutritionist. These professionals can make unique recommendations based on your needs, preferences, and health goals. They can help you develop a realistic and sustainable meal plan, identify areas for improvement in your diet, and provide Support and accountability as you work toward your weight loss objectives.

Seeking professional advice is important to ensure that your weight loss journey is effective and sustainable. Here's why getting advice from a qualified dietitian or nutritionist can be useful:

1. A trained dietitian or nutritionist: can make specialized suggestions based on your unique needs, preferences, and health goals. They will consider your age, gender, exercise level, medical history, and dietary preferences to develop a personalized meal plan that fits your nutritional needs while supporting your weight loss goals.

2. Evidence-Based Advice: Nutrition specialists make recommendations based on scientific evidence and current nutrition and dietetic research. They can help you distinguish between nutrition myths and fad diets, giving you accurate and dependable information to guide your dietary choices and lifestyle behaviours.

3. Accountability and Support: Working with a qualified dietitian or nutritionist ensures accountability and Support throughout your weight loss journey. They can help you create realistic objectives, track progress, and adjust your diet plan. A skilled and supportive professional can boost your motivation and confidence as you strive for your goals.

4. Behavioral therapy: In addition to nutrition guidance, registered dietitians and nutritionists are trained to provide behavioral therapy to assist you in developing healthy eating habits and overcoming barriers to your success. They can help you identify triggers for problematic eating behaviors, develop coping techniques for cravings and emotional eating, and implement long-term behaviour changes that promote weight maintenance.

5. Long-Term Success: By working with a nutrition professional, you can gain the information, skills, and habits required for long-term weight management and health improvement. They can provide the tools and information you need to make smart food choices, navigate social settings, and maintain healthy behaviours long after you've met your weight loss objectives.

Chapter 8.. Maintaining Progress and Long-Term Success

Maintaining development and attaining long-term success is the ultimate goal of every wellness program. In this chapter, we'll look at tactics and recommendations to help you keep your progress and continue your journey to health and wellbeing.

8. 1. Reflect on your journey.

Reflect on how far you've gone since starting your wellness journey. Celebrate your accomplishments, large and small, and recognize your obstacles. Recognizing your achievements and learning from your experiences can provide useful insights into what techniques worked best for you and which areas may require additional focus.

Reflecting on your wellness journey is an effective personal growth and development technique. It's about pausing, looking back, and appreciating how far you've come from the beginning. Here's why it matters:

1. Celebrating Successes: Recognizing your accomplishments, no matter how minor, is critical to retaining motivation and Momentum. Celebrate your accomplishments, such as sticking to an exercise schedule, eating healthier, or recognizing changes in your energy and attitude. Celebrating your triumphs reinforces positive behavior and boosts confidence in your capacity to attain your goals.

2. Learning from Challenges: You've likely met roadblocks and setbacks. Reflecting on these problems provides useful insights into what went wrong and why. Did you need help to maintain consistency in your workouts? Did stress or emotional eating disrupt your progress? By identifying the triggers and patterns that drive these issues, you may devise ways to overcome them in the future. Every setback presents a chance for development and learning.

3. Identifying Effective tactics: Reflecting on your journey allows you to identify the most effective tactics in helping you achieve your goals. You may have discovered that scheduling workouts in the morning improved your consistency or that food planning on weekends made it simpler to keep to a healthy diet during the week. By recognizing these great tactics, you can build on what works and improve your approach to achieve even better results.

4. Addressing Areas for Improvement: Reflecting on your journey might help you identify areas where you need to make improvements. You may need to pay more attention to your stress-management techniques or notice increased portion sizes. By identifying these areas for improvement, you can make proactive efforts to fix them and keep them from impeding your progress in the future.

Overall, reflecting on your wellness path promotes self-awareness, thankfulness, and resilience. It's about acknowledging how far you've come, learning from your experiences, and applying that information to keep moving toward your goals. So, take a minute to halt, reflect, and enjoy your accomplishments on the path to health and wellness.

8.2. Set Realistic Goals.

Creating realistic and attainable goals consistent with your long-term vision for health and wellbeing is critical as you progress. Break down your ambitions into smaller, more doable tasks that you can achieve gradually. Setting clear and attainable goals to improve your nutritional habits, increase your physical activity, or improve your stress management strategies will keep you motivated and focused on your trip.

Setting realistic goals is similar to constructing a road plan for your wellness journey. It is about setting clear, attainable goals to move you toward your long-term vision of health and wellbeing. Here's why it matters:

1. Aligning with Your Vision: Your objectives should reflect your overall vision for your health and wellbeing. Take some time to clarify your goals and why they are important. Your goals, whether to lose weight, improve fitness, reduce stress, or increase energy, should be consistent with your overall vision for a healthier lifestyle.

2. Breaking It Down: Once you have a clear idea, divide it into smaller, more achievable phases. These mini-goals serve as milestones on your journey, allowing you to monitor your progress and celebrate your accomplishments. Breaking down huge goals into smaller steps makes them less intimidating and more manageable.

3. Maintaining Motivation: Setting realistic goals helps you stay motivated and focused on your quest. When your goals are reachable, you're more likely to stick with your wellness regimen and persevere in the face of obstacles. Each minor win boosts your confidence and motivates you toward your greater goals.

4. Setting realistic goals enables incremental advancement and long-term Change. Instead of completely restructuring your lifestyle overnight, focus on making small changes over time. This technique helps you to gradually develop healthy behaviors, enhancing your chances of long-term success.

5. Adaptability: Realistic goals are adaptive to changing circumstances and priorities. Life is unpredictable, and unforeseen hurdles can develop along the path. Setting flexible goals allows you to change your approach without becoming discouraged or overwhelmed.

6. Focusing Your Efforts: Setting clear, attainable goals helps to guide and focus your efforts. They assist you in prioritizing your time, energy, and resources, ensuring that they are invested in the areas that will most influence your overall well being.

Remember that developing realistic goals involves striking a balance between ambition and achievability. Aim high, but consider what is realistically possible given your situation, resources, and restrictions. Setting clear, attainable goals, breaking them down into small steps, and remaining committed to your path can put you on track to achieving your vision of health and wellbeing.

8. 3. Stay Consistent.

Consistency is essential for making development and attaining long-term success. Commit to adopting healthy habits into your daily routine, whether doing chair yoga, eating nutritious meals, staying hydrated, or managing stress. Consistency builds habit, and you'll lay the groundwork for long-term success by including healthy choices in your daily routine.

Consistency is what ties your wellness journey together. It's about consistently showing up for yourself and making healthy choices in your daily routine. Here's why consistency is essential for advancement and long-term success:

1. Building Habits: Consistency is essential for habit building. When you repeat healthy activities, such as chair yoga, eating nutritious meals, and staying hydrated, you reinforce neural pathways in your brain that make those actions habitual. Over time, these habits become embedded in your daily routine, making it simpler to maintain your wellness goals without relying on willpower.

2. Creating Momentum: Consistent activity generates Momentum, propelling you forward in your journey. Each healthy choice you make builds on the previous one, causing a beneficial ripple effect throughout your life. As you accrue tiny victories and see progress over time, you'll acquire confidence in your ability to stay on track and meet your objectives.

3. Preventing Setbacks: Consistency is a buffer against potential setbacks and roadblocks along the path. When healthy habits are thoroughly embedded in your routine, you are better prepared to face challenges without derailing your progress. Consistency helps you stay grounded and focused on your long-term goals, even during stress or disturbance.

4. Cultivating Discipline: Consistency builds discipline, teaching you to prioritize your health and wellbeing even when difficult or inconvenient. It's about establishing a commitment to yourself and sticking to it daily, regardless of what happens around you. Over time, this discipline will become second nature, allowing you to overcome hurdles and stay the course.

5. Sustaining Progress: Long-term progress requires consistency. While quick-fix remedies may produce momentary improvements, long-term Change necessitates consistent effort and commitment. Sticking to your healthy habits provides the groundwork for future growth and improvement, ensuring that your progress is long-term and sustainable.

Incorporating healthy habits into your daily routine may not always be spectacular or exciting, but regular, small acts taken over time contribute to long-term transformation. So stay the course, be persistent, and believe in the ability of your daily routines to move you toward your long-term wellness goals.

8. 4. Prioritize self-care.

Self-care is critical to overall wellbeing but is sometimes forgotten when pursuing health and fitness goals. Make time for activities that benefit your mind, body, and spirit, such as taking a relaxing bath, engaging in a hobby, spending time with loved ones, or getting enough sleep. Prioritizing self-care will allow you to rest and regenerate, giving you the energy and resilience to keep up with your wellness goals.

Prioritizing self-care is similar to permitting yourself to refill your cup so you may continue pouring into others and pursuing your goals with vigor. Here's why it matters:

1. Nourishing Mind, Body, and Soul: Self-care activities nourish all aspects of your being, including physical, emotional, and spiritual. Whether taking a bubble bath, practicing mindfulness meditation, or spending quality time with loved ones, these activities restore your energy reserves and improve your overall wellness.

2. Preventing Burnout: In today's fast-paced world, it's easy to become engrossed in the hustle and bustle of daily life, often at the expense of our health. Prioritizing self-care provides a protective buffer against burnout and tiredness. You may avoid stress and maintain a healthy work-life balance by scheduling time for relaxation and rejuvenation.

3. Self-care promotes resilience: the ability to recover from misfortune and thrive in the face of adversities. When you prioritize self-care, you develop emotional and physical resilience, giving yourself the resources to deal with stressors and disappointments. As a result, you can handle life's ups and downs with grace and perseverance.

4. Improving Mental Health: Maintaining healthy mental health and emotional wellbeing requires prioritizing self-care. Activities that bring you joy, contentment, and relaxation might help you feel less stressed, anxious, and depressed. Taking a nature walk, writing your thoughts and feelings, or practicing gratitude are all examples of self-care techniques that improve mood and create inner calm.

5. Increasing Productivity and Creativity: Self-care is strategic; unlike common assumptions, self-care is not selfish. When you prioritize self-care, you replenish your batteries and sharpen your cognitive abilities, increasing attention, productivity, and creativity. Regular breaks to rest and refresh improve your long-term effectiveness and efficiency because you approach jobs with renewed vigor and clarity.

self-care promotes self-compassion—treating oneself with love, understanding, and acceptance, particularly during adversity or failure. Prioritizing self-care affirms your innate worth and value, realizing you deserve the same love, care, and attention as everyone else.

Incorporating self-care into your daily routine is not a luxury but essential for long-term health and wellbeing. Make self-care a non-negotiable element of your daily routine, and watch as your physical, mental, and emotional health improves. Remember, you can't pour from an empty cup, so prioritize self-care and replenish your reserves regularly.

8. 5. Monitor your progress.

Monitor your progress regularly to see where you stand and where you can improve. Keep a notebook to track your workouts, food, feelings, and any obstacles you face. Tracking your progress shows how far you've gone and provides useful feedback for adjusting your strategy. Celebrate your accomplishments, and view setbacks as chances for growth and learning.

Monitoring your progress is like having a compass on your wellness journey—it helps you stay on track, overcome difficulties, and celebrate accomplishments. Here's why it matters:

1. Visibility and Accountability: Tracking your progress clearly shows where you stand regarding your goals. Keeping a journal provides physical documentation of your efforts and triumphs, whether for tracking your exercises, food intake, or emotions. This visibility makes you accountable to yourself, ensuring that you stick to your goals even when things go rough.

2. Identifying Patterns and Trends: By tracking your progress, you can identify patterns and trends that may influence your success. By tracking variables like exercise frequency, eating habits, mood swings, and energy levels, you can determine which aspects help or impede your success. This knowledge enables you to make informed decisions and modifications to improve your outcomes.

3. Motivation and Encouragement: Seeing visible results of your efforts may be extremely inspiring and encouraging. Whether you notice increases in your strength, endurance, mood, or favorable changes in your body composition or health markers, recognizing these accomplishments enhances your confidence and reaffirms your dedication to your goals. Furthermore, focusing on how far you've come might help you stay inspired throughout difficult times and remind you of your strength and determination.

4. Course Correction and Adaptation: Tracking your progress provides useful data that allows you to change your strategy as necessary. Run into roadblocks or setbacks along the way, such as weight loss plateaus or motivation drops. Examining your notebook can help you identify likely causes and build strategies to overcome them. Monitoring your progress allows you to make informed decisions and course corrections to stay on track toward your goals, whether adjusting your training regimen, fine-tuning your dietary plan, or implementing stress management tactics.

5. Cultivating Self-Awareness: Regularly assessing your progress promotes self-awareness—the ability to listen to your thoughts, feelings, and behaviors with curiosity and compassion. Observing how different circumstances affect your wellbeing and performance helps you better understand your habits, triggers, and behavioral patterns. This self-awareness creates the groundwork for personal development and transformation, allowing you to make deliberate decisions that are consistent with your beliefs and goals.

Incorporating progress monitoring into your wellness journey is more than just tracking numbers; it's about better understanding yourself and your path. So take a diary, start charting your progress, and watch as it transforms into a powerful instrument for personal growth, empowerment, and long-term improvement. Remember that every stride forward, no matter how tiny, is a step closer to becoming your best self.

8. 6. Stay Flexible and Adaptable.

Life is full of surprises, and keeping up needs flexibility and adaptability. Be willing to adapt your goals and techniques as circumstances change and new obstacles emerge. Feel free to try something different if you need a different strategy. Remain resilient in the face of failures, and remember that they are only temporary roadblocks on the way to long-term achievement.

Staying flexible and adaptable is similar to being a skillful navigator on the ever-changing seas of life—it allows you to change direction and handle adversities with grace and perseverance. Here's why it matters:

1. Embracing Change: Life is inherently unpredictable, and making progress necessitates a willingness to adapt to changing conditions. Whether it's a change in your job schedule, your health, or unforeseen occurrences that disturb your routine, remaining flexible helps you roll with the punches and alter your objectives and methods as needed. Embracing Change rather than opposing it allows you to manage life's twists and turns with greater ease and resilience.

2. Experimentation and Innovation: Adaptability allows you to explore new ways and strategies to attain your objectives. Feel free to try something new if a specific workout program or food plan needs to produce the intended results. Experiment with activities, food plans, and lifestyle behaviors to determine best. You can find inventive solutions that propel you to success by remaining open-minded and willing to explore new options.

3. Resilience in the Face of Setbacks: Setbacks are unavoidable in any journey, but how you handle them defines your final success. Staying flexible and adaptive helps you develop resilience—the ability to recover from adversity and emerge stronger. When faced with setbacks or hurdles, see them as opportunities for growth and learning, not impenetrable barriers. Adjust your strategy, learn from your mistakes, and use setbacks as stepping stones to move you forward in your quest.

4. Maintaining Momentum: Being flexible and adaptive allows you to keep Momentum on your path to advancement and achievement. Rather than being discouraged by failures or challenges, utilize them as motivation to move forward. Even when faced with difficulties, you can keep progressing steadily toward your goals by remaining adaptable and altering your approach as needed. Remember that growth is not always linear, and setbacks are a normal part of the process. Stay flexible and resilient, and keep pushing forward one step at a time.

5. Empowerment and Self-Trust: Finally, remaining flexible and adaptable allows you to take control of your trip and believe in your ability to overcome problems. By accepting Change and keeping open to new opportunities, you display perseverance, resourcefulness, and self-confidence. Trust yourself to manage life's uncertainties with grace and resilience, knowing you are flexible and adaptable enough to face any difficulty.

Incorporating flexibility and adaptation into your advancement strategy ensures you can confidently and resiliently negotiate life's twists and turns. Accept Change, remain open-minded, and believe in your ability to overcome challenges, recognizing that adaptability is the key to long-term progress and success.

Chapter 9

28-Days Rapid Weight lose Challenge

Day 1: Chair Yoga Introduction

- Begin by sitting comfortably in a sturdy chair, feet flat on the ground and spine upright.

- Close your eyes and take several deep breaths, in through your nose and out through your mouth.

- Set your challenge goals: enhance your health, increase mobility, and reduce weight swiftly through gentle chair yoga exercises.

- Let's start with your eyes open!

Day 2: Gentle Warm Up

- Sit tall in your chair, hands on your knees.

- Take deep breaths, extending your spine and raising your chest.

- Exhale slowly, rounding your back and lowering your chin to your chest.

- Do this seated cat-cow stretch five times, focusing on the movement of your spine and the rhythm of your breath.

Day 3: Sitting Sun Salutations

- Inhale and bring your arms up, palms contacting.

- Exhale and lower your hands to your heart.

- Repeat this pattern five times, following your breath and feeling the energy flow through your body.

Day 4: Chair Forward Bend

- Inhale deeply while stretching your spine.

- Exhale, pivot at the hips and bend forward to reach your feet.

- Hold for 15 seconds, feeling the stretch in your hamstrings and lower back.

- Inhale as you slowly return to a sitting position.

Day 5: Seated Spinal Twist

-Inhale and straighten your spine.

- Exhale and twist to the right, keeping your left hand on your right knee and your right hand on the back of the chair.

- Hold for 15 seconds, feeling the twist in your spine and opening in your chest.

- Inhale back into the center, then exhale and twist to the left, repeating on the opposite side.

Day Six: Chair Warrior II

- Inhale, stretch your arms to the sides, palms facing down.

- Exhale, then bend your right knee to align with your right ankle.

- Focus on your right fingertips to feel strong and anchored in your chair warrior II position.

- Hold on to this pose for about 15 seconds and switch sides.

Day Seven: Seated Tree Pose

- Inhale and lift your right foot off the ground, resting on your left inner thigh.

- Exhale and place your right foot against your left thigh, then your left thigh against your right.

- Hold your seated tree stance for 15 seconds to achieve balance and stability.

Repeat on the opposite side.

Day 8: Seated Warrior I.

- Sit upright in your chair, feet hip-width apart.

- Inhale, then extend your arms above, palms facing each other.

- Exhale, and then bend your right knee so that it is squarely over your right ankle.

- As you raise your arms, press down with your right foot to feel a stretch in your arms and legs.

- Hold for 15 seconds, then switch sides and repeat.

Day 9: Seated Side Stretch

- Sit tall on your chair, feet flat on the ground.

- Inhale and extend your right arm above, stretching your side body.

- Exhale, then gradually bend to the left, feeling the strain on your right side.

- Hold for 15 seconds, then switch sides and repeat.

Day 10: Chair Mountain Pose

- Sit tall on your chair with your feet flat on the ground.

- Inhale deeply while bringing your arms up, palms facing each other.

- Exhale by pressing your palms together and engaging your core muscles.

- Hold for 20 seconds, feeling strong and steady as a mountain.

Day 11: Seated Forward Fold with Twist

- Sit upright with feet flat on the floor.

Inhale and straighten your spine.

- Exhale, pivot at the hips and bend forward to reach your feet.

- Inhale, then lengthen your spine again.

- Exhale and twist to the right, keeping your left hand on your right knee and your right hand on the back of the chair.

- Hold for 15 seconds, experiencing the stretch in your hamstrings and spine.

- Inhale back into the center, exhale, and twist to the left side.

Day 12: Seated Cat-Cow With Arm Extension

- Sit at the front edge of your chair, feet flat on the ground.

- Inhale, arch your back and raise your chest with your arms extended forward.

- Exhale, circle your spine and return your arms to your body.

- Repeat this pattern ten times, focusing on the movement of your spine and arms.

Day 13: Chair Warriors III

- Sit upright in your chair, feet hip-width apart.

- Inhale and raise your arms upwards.

- Exhale, hinge at the hips and lean forward with your left leg straight back.

- Keep your hips square, and your toes pointed at the ground.

- Hold for 15 seconds, then switch sides and repeat.

Day 14: The Seated Half Moon Pose.

- Sit tall on your chair with your feet flat on the ground.

- Inhale, extend your right arm overhead, reaching up and across to the left.

- Exhale, then gradually bend to the left, feeling the strain on your right side.

- Hold for 15 seconds, then switch sides and repeat.

Day 15: Seated Warriors' Flow

- Sit straight on your chair, feet flat on the ground.

- Inhale and raise your arms upwards.

- Exhale, bend your right elbow, bring it behind your head, then stretch your left arm to the floor.

- Inhale and then return to the center.

- Exhale, bend your left elbow behind your head, then extend your right arm downward.

- Continue the flowing action for ten rounds, focusing on the stretch in your side body.

Day 16: The Seated Chair Pose

 - Sit tall with feet hip-width apart.

Inhale, then raise your arms upwards.

- Exhale while bending your knees and lowering your hips as if you were sitting on an unseen chair.

- Hold for 15 seconds, keeping your weight on your heels and your spine long.

Day 17: Seated Twist with Leg Extension.

- Sit upright in your chair and flat your feet on the floor.

- Inhale and straighten your spine.

- Exhale and twist to the right, keeping your left hand on your right knee and your right hand on the back of the chair.

- Inhale and then extend your left leg out to the side.

- Exhale and bring your navel inside, towards your spine, feeling the stretch in your spine and outer hip.

- Hold for 15 seconds, then switch sides and repeat.

Day 18: Seated Side Bend with Arm Reach.

- Sit upright in your chair and place your feet flat on the floor.

- Inhale and raise your right arm above, lengthening your side body.

- Exhale, then gradually bend to the left, feeling the strain on your right side.

Inhale, raise your left arm overhead, then bend to the right.

- Exhale and feel the stretch on your left side.

- Repeat this side-to-side movement ten times, letting your breath flow.

Day 19: Seated Eagle Arms

- Sit upright in your chair and place your feet flat on the floor.

- Inhale and spread your arms to the sides.

- Exhale and cross your right arm over your left, wrapping your forearms and possibly bringing your hands together.

- Raise your elbows slightly and hold for 15 seconds to experience a stretch between your shoulder blades.

- Let go and switch sides, crossing your left arm over the right.

Day 20: Seated Figure Four Stretch

- Sit erect on your chair, feet flat on the ground.

- Cross your right ankle over your left knee while flexing your right foot to protect the knee joint.

Inhale and straighten your spine.

- Exhale, then gently press down on your right knee to feel a stretch in your outer hip.

- Hold for 15 seconds, then switch sides and repeat.

Day 21: Seated Mountain Pose with Shoulder Rolls.

- Sit tall, and place your feet flat on the ground.

- Inhale and bring your shoulders up to your ears.

- Exhale and move your shoulders back and down, feeling the space in your chest.

- Repeat this shoulder roll for ten rounds, focusing on releasing tension in your shoulders and upper back.

Day 22: Seated Side Leg Lifts.

- Sit upright on your chair, feet flat on the ground and hands resting on your hips.

Inhale and straighten your spine.

- Exhale, engage your core, and lift your right leg to the side, keeping it straight.

- Pause briefly at the apex, then inhale and lower your leg.

- Continue along the left side.

- Repeat for ten reps on each side, focusing on controlled motions and strengthening your outer thigh muscles.

Day 23: Seated Boat Pose

- Sit at the front edge of your chair, feet flat on the ground and knees bent.

- Place your hands lightly on the sides of the chair to provide further support.

- Inhale, stretch your back, and raise your feet, bringing your shins parallel to the floor.

- Engage your core muscles to maintain balance.

- Hold a steady breathing rate for 10-15 seconds.

- Exhale as you return your feet to the ground.

- Repeat 3-5 times, gradually increasing hold time as your strength improves.

Day 24: Seated Shoulder Openers

- Sit erect in your chair, feet level with the ground.

- Interlace your fingers behind your back, extend your arms, and squeeze your shoulder blades together.

- Inhale, raise your chest, and slightly lean your head back to allow air to flow through the front of your body.

- Hold for 15 to 30 seconds, taking deep breaths and feeling the stretch in your chest and shoulders.

- Exhale as you exit the position and place your hands in your lap.

- Repeat 2-3 times, aiming to increase the stretch with each breath.

Day 25: Seated Knee to Chest Stretch.

- Sit at the front edge of your chair with your feet flat on the ground.

- For support, grab the chair's sides.

- Inhale, bring your right knee to your chest, and clutch it with your hands.

- Hold for 10-15 seconds, experiencing a stretch in your hips and lower back.

- Exhale as you drop your leg.

- Continue along the left side.

- Continue to do 8-10 repetitions on each side, moving with your breath and maintaining appropriate posture.

Day 26: Seated Cat-Cow with Leg Extension.

 - Sit facing the front edge of your chair, feet flat on the ground.

- Put your hands on your knees.

- Inhale, arch your back, and elevate your chest, extending your right leg in front of you.

- Exhale, circle your spine and bring your knee back to your chest.

- Continue along the left side.

- Repeat the cat-cow and leg extension exercises ten times on each side, moving with your breath and concentrating on the suppleness of your spine.

Day 27: Seated Side Plank.

- Sit at the front edge of your chair and place your feet flat on the floor.

- Place your right hand on the chair seat, fingers pointing toward you.

- Inhale and lift your hips off the chair, stretching your legs to the sides and stacking your feet.

- Raise your left arm to the ceiling, making a straight line from your heels to your fingertips.

- Hold 10-15 seconds while engaging your core and elevating your hips.

- Exhale as you lower your hips back into the chair.

- Continue along the left side.

- Continue to alternate between right and left side planks for 3-5 repetitions per side, focusing on stability and control.

Day 28: Seated Relaxation

- Sit comfortably in your chair, feet flat on the ground, and hands on your lap.

- Close your eyes and take deep breaths through your nose and mouth.

- Allow your body to relax fully, letting go of all tension and stress.

- Stay in this seated relaxation pose for 5-10 minutes, concentrating on your breathing and allowing yourself to relax fully.

- When ready, gently open your eyes and bring your attention back to the present moment.

Congratulations on completing the 28-day guided challenge for rapid weight loss with chair yoga! Remember to listen to your body, alter the positions as necessary, and reap the benefits of improved fitness and well-being. Keep up the great work!

Conclusion

As we conclude our trip through "Chair Yoga for Seniors to Lose Weight," I'd want to convey my heartfelt gratitude for joining me on this revolutionary path to health and well-being. Throughout this book, we've looked at the powerful intersection of chair yoga, nutrition, and mindful living, uncovering the secrets to long-term weight loss and overall wellness.

As we've learned, chair yoga is a gentle yet effective way for seniors to increase mobility, strength, and general fitness—all from the comfort of their own chair. By introducing basic yet effective yoga poses, breathing techniques, and relaxation exercises into your daily routine, you are taking a proactive approach to reclaiming your health and energy.

But chair yoga is only one part of the puzzle. We've also discussed the significance of nutrition, emphasizing the benefits of a well-balanced diet rich in whole foods, portion control, and mindful eating habits. By fueling your body with nutrient-dense foods and staying hydrated, you establish the framework for long-term weight loss and good health.

Aside from the physical factors, we've investigated the enormous impact of mentality, self-care, and thankfulness on your wellness path. Cultivating a happy outlook, prioritizing self-care, and practicing appreciation for the benefits in your life all contribute to your mental and emotional well-being, which are critical components of overall health.

As you continue on your path to health and vitality, keep in mind that progress is not always linear, and setbacks are inevitable. Accept the trip with respect and compassion for yourself, appreciating your accomplishments and learning from setbacks along the way.

Finally, I want to encourage you to apply the principles and practices contained in this book as you continue on your wellness path. Whether you want to lose a few pounds, increase your mobility, or simply improve your general well-being, remember that you have the ability to effect positive change in your life.

Thank you for choosing me as your guide on this adventure. May your road be full with joy, vitality, and good health. Here's to a vibrant, fulfilling life propelled by the transformational power of chair yoga and mindfulness. Continue to shine brightly, and may your journey be filled with abundant health, pleasure, and tranquility.

With thanks and kindest wishes,

[Daniel S. Leeper]

CHAIR YOGA FOR SENIORS TO LOSE WEIGHT 

WEEKLY
PLANNER

Monday	Tuesday	Wednesday

Thursday	Friday	Saturday

Sunday	Important Notes:
	....

WEEKLY
PLANNER

Monday

Tuesday

Wednesday

Thursday

Friday

Saturday

Sunday

Important Notes:

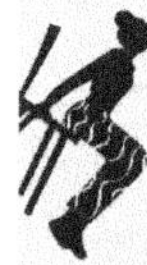

WEEKLY
PLANNER

Monday

Tuesday

Wednesday

Thursday

Friday

Saturday

Sunday

Important Notes:

....

....

....

....

....

 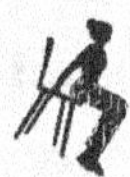

WEEKLY
PLANNER

Monday	Tuesday	Wednesday

Thursday	Friday	Saturday

Sunday

Important Notes:

....
....
....
....
....

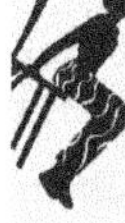

WEEKLY
PLANNER

Monday	Tuesday	Wednesday

Thursday	Friday	Saturday

Sunday	Important Notes:
	....

WEEKLY
PLANNER

Monday	Tuesday	Wednesday

Thursday	Friday	Saturday

Sunday	Important Notes:
	....

 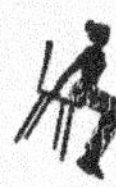

WEEKLY
PLANNER

Monday

Tuesday

Wednesday

Thursday

Friday

Saturday

Sunday

Important Notes:

....

....

....

....

....

WEEKLY
PLANNER

Monday	Tuesday	Wednesday

Thursday	Friday	Saturday

Sunday	Important Notes:

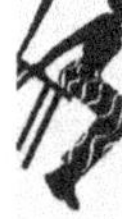

 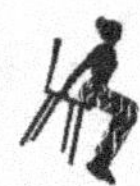

WEEKLY
PLANNER

Monday

Tuesday

Wednesday

Thursday

Friday

Saturday

Sunday

Important Notes:

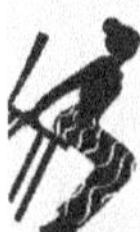

WEEKLY
PLANNER

Monday

Tuesday

Wednesday

Thursday

Friday

Saturday

Sunday

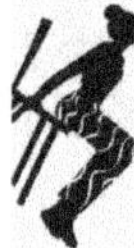

Important Notes:

....

....

....

....

....

 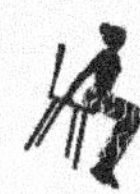

WEEKLY
PLANNER

Monday	Tuesday	Wednesday

Thursday	Friday	Saturday

Sunday	Important Notes:
	....
	....
	....
	....
	....

WEEKLY
PLANNER

Monday	Tuesday	Wednesday

Thursday	Friday	Saturday

Sunday	Important Notes:
	....

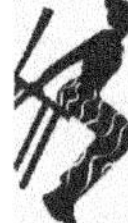

WEEKLY
PLANNER

Monday	Tuesday	Wednesday
Thursday	Friday	Saturday

Sunday	Important Notes:

 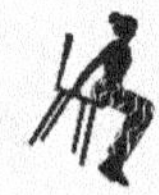

WEEKLY
PLANNER

Monday	Tuesday	Wednesday
Thursday	Friday	Saturday

Sunday	Important Notes:

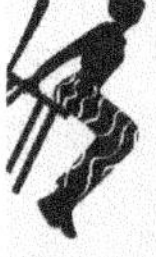

 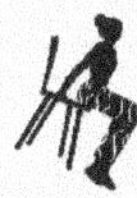

WEEKLY
PLANNER

Monday	Tuesday	Wednesday

Thursday	Friday	Saturday

Sunday	Important Notes:

WEEKLY
PLANNER

Monday

Tuesday

Wednesday

Thursday

Friday

Saturday

Sunday

Important Notes:

....

....

....

....

....

WEEKLY
PLANNER

Monday	Tuesday	Wednesday
Thursday	Friday	Saturday
Sunday	Important Notes:	

WEEKLY
PLANNER

Monday	Tuesday	Wednesday
Thursday	Friday	Saturday

Sunday	Important Notes:

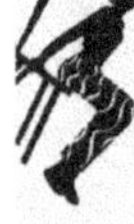

WEEKLY
PLANNER

Monday

Tuesday

Wednesday

Thursday

Friday

Saturday

Sunday

Important Notes:

....

....

....

....

....

WEEKLY
PLANNER

Monday	Tuesday	Wednesday

Thursday	Friday	Saturday

Sunday	Important Notes:
	....
	....
	....
	....
	....

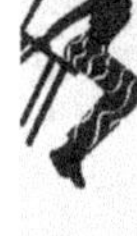

www.ingramcontent.com/pod-product-compliance
Lightning Source LLC
Chambersburg PA
CBHW081220260726
48653CB00010BB/3705